M000316498

HOT MESS TO WELLNESS

AMANDA L. ZEINE, DO, FAAP

HOT MESS
TO
Wellness

7 Steps to Better Health When You Have Tried It All and Had Enough

AMANDA L. ZEINE, DO, FAAP

ISBN paperback: 978-1-7378412-0-3
ISBN E-book: 978-1-7378412-1-0

I dedicate this book to my daughter. You will always be my baby, even as you grow into a strong independent young woman. Shoot for the stars, kiddo. You can do anything. I love you.

READ THIS FIRST

As a thank you for purchasing *Hot Mess to Wellness*, I'm gifting you a copy of my Wellness Journey Log. *Visit https://www.hot-mess-to-wellness.com/copy-of-resources* to download your free copy. While there, explore the blog and forum of people who are also on a journey from hot mess to wellness. As a community we can support one another as we travel this journey.

WELLNESS JOURNEY
WEEKLY LOG

CONTENTS

INTRODUCTION

I have teetered on the line of being normal weight and overweight since my early twenties, yet it became a growing issue (no pun intended) once I passed thirty-five. If you know anything about the military, you understand that weight is watched closely. They require us to have our height and weight recorded twice yearly, and if we're overweight we have to be "taped." This measures our body fat content. They have always required me to be taped because of my weight teetering on the line. And that was all despite the fact that I was a fairly healthy person who exercised a few times a week and ate healthy foods.

In April 2021, though, I reached my heaviest weight—187 pounds (body mass index of 32). I was beside myself. This was one pound heavier than my weight at nine months pregnant. I had become *obese*! It's not like this happened overnight. The struggle with being borderline had finally tipped me into another level of being officially classified as obese!

How did this happen? Well, looking back, I had really been obese for about two years but was reluctant to admit it. In December 2018, I had a fall resulting in a traumatic brain injury (TBI). At the time, I was a Major in the United States Army, thriving in my career as a pediatrician. After my injury, I had significant symptoms requiring brain rest. I could not drive or work.

Then there I was two years later and at my heaviest. I blamed my weight gain on my head injury, depression, medication changes, migraines...the list goes on. As my husband would say, I am the "Queen of Rationalization."

When I hit that shocking number in 2021 it was time I stopped rationalizing and admitted the truth: "I am obese because I eat too much, have minimal will power, and am not moving enough to burn the calories I am eating." Not only was I obese, I was also sluggish despite using my CPAP (continuous positive airway pressure) machine for sleep apnea. I felt unmotivated to do much of anything, especially exercise. *Why was it so difficult to live a "normal life" and feel healthy?*

Throughout my life I had tried many of the fad diets and failed, the result was always me gaining back the weight lost, plus some. I paid astronomical amounts of money to have procedures done to help me look thinner and kill off fat cells. None of these worked and just wasted my hard-earned money.

Why did I do these things? I wanted something easy to help me lose weight because I thought losing weight would make me feel better physically and emotionally. *If I felt better, I would be motivated to eat right and exercise, right?*

Wrong!

Being a physician who has counseled many overweight patients, I knew what to do. I knew I was doing all the wrong things, and that there was no magic solution. I just didn't have the motivation to do the right things or the patience to put in the work to build the needed good habits. Unfortunately I was the only one who could change any of this. I decided enough was enough! No more fad diets, supplements, gym memberships, and most of all, denial of my obesity. I decided it was time to accept my diagnosis and motivate myself to do something about it.

Society's trend toward obesity because of suboptimal wellness is a significant problem. Compounding that problem are our societal tendencies to want a quick fix using fad diets and supplements, which only leads to failure and feeling worse.

In this book, I want to show you why being "skinny" is not necessarily healthy or true wellness. I am sharing my story so you can see that you are not alone in this journey. There are many people in this world who struggle as they age—it's tough to stay healthy and/ or to achieve optimal wellness. Our fast-paced life and the constant feelings of limited time make us stuck in our ways. I want to show you what wellness truly is and how simple it can be to achieve.

But what is optimal wellness? *Optimal wellness* is the state in which you feel well, are free of disease and injury, and have peace of mind. In this state you do not have chronic fatigue and grogginess, you have the energy and motivation to get up and get moving, you eat healthy whole foods that fuel your body, and you are truly happy.

In my own journey, I discovered what I refer to as the Seven Pillars of Optimal Wellness. These are so simple to incorporate into your life. Throughout this book, you will learn how to be mindful and relax, and how to revise your habits to improve sleep. You'll learn the importance of hydration and eating healthy foods (and what *not* to eat). You'll also discover that exercise does not have to be intense to be right for you, and that having a support system is important to stay motivated.

Only you can take charge and find your optimal wellness. Once you incorporate these Seven Pillars of Optimal Wellness into your routine, you'll notice that your clothes seem to fit better, you'll lose inches, and you'll begin to feel less fatigued. These Seven Pillars will not only lead to your optimal wellness but also build the habits to easily sustain it.

I will walk with you as you find the motivation to tackle each obstacle. I recommend you start by reading one chapter at a time and incorporating that pillar into your routine before moving on to the next. To help you along the way, check out the material on my website *https://www.hot-mess-to-wellness.com/*. Let's get this party started!

Chapter 1

MINDFULNESS

"BE HAPPY IN THE MOMENT, THAT'S ENOUGH. EACH MOMENT IS ALL WE
NEED, NOT MORE." -MOTHER TERESA

I have never been great at living in the moment. As an Army physician, I climbed my way up to the position of Chief of Pediatrics at an Army community hospital. I have worked both as a provider in the outpatient clinic and in the inpatient mother-baby unit, all while attending meetings and overseeing all pediatric operations. Sometimes I worked the day shift, sometimes night, and sometimes the night shift lengthened into the day because of meetings. Bottom line is…I worked *a lot*!

I had a horrible work-life balance, and all I knew was go, go, go. Then in December 2018 my life changed in an instant when I suffered a traumatic brain injury (TBI). When I fell, I ignored all the signs of a concussion and continued working. Working unfortunately worsened all of my symptoms.

Due to the seriousness of my condition, I could not drive for over six weeks. I was alone because my husband had deployed five days after my injury, and my daughter and stepsons were with their other respective parents. Once I listened to others and took time for myself, I realized how bad my symptoms really were.

Daily migraines and headaches continued from the head injury.

I slept a lot and had no focus or purpose. I had every delivery app known to man on my phone and ate my feelings away if I wasn't sleeping. I was not mindful of my feelings or being fully present in my life.

After two months of minimal improvement, my neurologist referred me to the Traumatic Brain Injury Clinic. And part of my recovery was seeing a psychologist. While going through therapy, I realized a core part of my problem was my loss of identity. I had once been a successful physician and Army officer, and now I was a *hot mess*. I had many physical and emotional issues to deal with, but I needed to learn how to accept who I was at that moment. I needed to learn how to appreciate the past but accept myself for the person I had become. *But how?*

I used to think the people talking about being mindful were absurd. Get up early and take the time to reflect—blah, blah, blah. I was too busy for that stuff. I was working long hours, sometimes even on different shifts. *Who has time to get up early to do that crap?*

If this head injury has taught me anything, it was that burnout is real. Looking back, the "old me" was on the path to burnout. The "new me" decided maybe I should give this mindfulness stuff a chance.

Through my recovery program at the TBI clinic, I was enrolled in a mindful meditation program. I saw benefits almost immediately. Meditation did not lessen my headaches, but it helped me to let go of my stress, even if only for the twenty to thirty minutes I was in the class. It was then that I realized the importance of mindfulness. It became an integral part of my plan that later developed into my Seven Pillars of Optimal Wellness.

After that success I went out and bought multiple books about meditation. I then thought maybe I should try crystals and essential oils. I bought so many things that I thought would help me with my experience. Note that if you feel crystals and essential oils help with your practice, I am not judging you. It's just that none of it worked for me and ended up being more money wasted.

I'm here to tell all of you that it takes nothing physical to practice mindfulness or meditation. You just need to learn to focus your mind and learn how to live in the present.

Easier said than done, I know.

WHAT IS MINDFULNESS?

Merriam-Webster.com defines *mindfulness* as "the practice of maintaining a nonjudgmental state of heightened or complete awareness of one's thoughts, emotions, or experiences on a moment-to-moment basis."[1]

There are many ways to be mindful including but not limited to practicing meditation, giving up the need for perfectionism, allowing yourself to no longer focus on control of those things for which you have no control, or being present in the moment. One can simply try to live a good life, be nonjudgmental, live in the present, and have appropriate expectations of themselves and others. Again, easier said than done.

Humans are naturally judgmental beings. We need consistency to refocus ourselves and form good habits. Once we form these good habits, we can release those bad habits of being judgmental, being a perfectionist, and holding grudges. We need to learn to let things go.

We also need to learn not only to be kind to others but also to ourselves. One way to do that is to get into a consistent routine of practicing mindfulness daily. It can be as simple as a routine that only takes about five to ten minutes first thing every morning; practicing this before you start the day can make a tremendous difference in how you perceive the day's events. Such a routine helps you to slow down. Slowing down reduces stress, and you perceive things in a more positive light. Less stress is one thing we as a society desperately need so we can improve our overall health and wellness.

My typical morning previously involved hitting the snooze button at least two to three times, then jumping out of bed thinking, *Oh crap, I'm late!* I would pour a cup of coffee in a travel mug as I was running out the door.

That, my friend, is not the right way to start your morning mindfully. Now I try to wake up at least thirty minutes earlier. With that extra time, I can take the morning more slowly, get a cup of coffee, and sit down to relax. Now I don't feel rushed, and my day starts out with less stress. I leave knowing I have plenty of time to get wherever I am going and with time to spare. Being mindful can be as simple as slowing down and allowing yourself time to live in the present, but I recommend diving deeper.

A daily mindfulness practice helps even more than just slowing down. At the end of this chapter, I will show you one simple exercise. And to learn more, you can visit my website *https://www.hot-mess-to-wellness.com/*.

THERE'S MORE TO BEING MINDFUL

Please understand that there is more to being mindful than just doing a simple exercise a few minutes a day. Unfortunately other things sometimes can pull us out of the present and create barriers to us being mindful. Perfectionism, high expectations of ourselves and others, and procrastination are just a few. These three things can cause significant added stress and definitely hinder your ability to be mindful and live in the present.

For instance, being a type A personality and constantly striving for perfection in my everyday life led me to many letdowns time after time. The disappointment and stress I had with each let down just added to my already troublesome life.

The "old me" was constantly pushing myself to be perfect. And because of that I would sometimes procrastinate doing things because I didn't have the time to make the finished product perfect. The "new me" has learned that everything in life is not perfect, and we cannot plan our lives. We are on a path that we don't always have control over, and there will be times we need to let go of our need for perfectionism and control, and be mindful of the things we can control in this moment. Again, easier said than done. Just trust that it *can* be done.

When you're feeling overwhelmed by procrastination or the need for perfection, it's time to stop and take a time out. I know you are thinking, *What? Time out! I am not five!* But even as an adult, you occasionally need to stop, take a time out, take a few deep breaths, and focus on what's really important.

Am I expecting more than I should of myself or someone else? Do I really have to plan that entire day down to the minute? Can I start that project knowing that if I work on it, I can fine tune things later?

Asking these questions has helped me to see that the world isn't perfect, I am not perfect, and I can lower my perfectionistic standards. Note that I'm not saying that you shouldn't have standards or that you should lower your standards in such a way that you don't produce quality work. I'm simply saying many of us are too hard on ourselves and others—and life doesn't have to be that way.

SELF-TALK

Self-talk is that inner voice talking to you, and it can be positive or negative. If you are like me, it is more negative than positive, causing you to be very hard on yourself. Negative self-talk is something we need to be mindful of and squash. The number one reason for negative self-talk in my opinion is comparing yourself to others. *Don't do it!*

Have you heard of cognitive distortions? *Cognitive distortions* are thoughts you have that are distorted and rooted in your deep inner values. They usually come from your subconscious, and you don't even realize you have them. They also lead to negative self-talk. Some cognitive distortions are listed below.

- **Polarized thinking**. This happens when you think in extremes such as "I am a complete failure."
- **Catastrophizing.** This occurs when you think the absolute worst, and when something small happens you spiral downward to the worst possible outcome.
- **Mind reading.** This happens when you assume you know what others are thinking, and it can increase anxiety.
- **Emotional reasoning.** This occurs when you have a false belief that what you feel is the truth, but when in reality it is not the truth.

This list is not all-inclusive, but these are a few I find myself falling into often. And they always cause worsening anxiety and worry. If you find yourself doing any of these you need to rethink the situation. If you can get into a mindful mental state, it is easier to recognize these as well.

When you find yourself needing a time out, *stop*, close your eyes, take those deep cleansing breaths, and be mindful. Do you have time for more than just a few deep breaths? Take it. The more time you attempt to spend in the present, the happier you will feel.

Remember that this is something that will need to be done consistently, and we all go through times where we are less dedicated. You may fall back into old habits. I have. We are all human and it happens. Just remember how simple this was to incorporate and jump back into it. As we near the end of this first pillar on our journey to wellness, I want to remind you that mindfulness can be easily achieved. It will take commitment, consistency, and perseverance on your part to let go of perfectionism, procrastination, judgment, worry, and overly high expectations.

Today is day one of your journey to optimal wellness, and today mindfulness is the top priority.

MINDFUL BREATHING

I would like to introduce you to an exercise in mindful breathing, which is a great mindfulness practice.

1. Find a quiet place and get comfortable. If you are more comfortable sitting, try to sit upright, and if on a chair, try to sit at the edge with both feet on the floor. If you choose to lie down, it is best to lie supine (on your back).
2. Close your eyes and clear your mind. Relax your body.
3. Now just breathe.

   • Breathe in through your nose. When breathing through the nose, nitric oxide in the air being breathed is increased, and this gas dilates vessels and helps to open the airways, allowing the lungs to have full capacity and more efficient oxygen exchange.

- Breathe out through your mouth to release toxins and carbon dioxide. Your exhaled breath should be about two times longer than your inhaled breath to help keep lungs expanded fully and for a longer time.
- Focus on the rhythm of your breathing.

4. Calm any internal monologue. You may notice your mind wandering. Refocus on your breathing.
5. Do this for five to ten minutes, refocusing if your mind wanders.

Try this and see how it makes you feel. You may find your mind wandering more in the beginning. As you continue to refocus your thoughts, maintaining your focus throughout the exercise should become easier.

MINDFULNESS USING THE FIVE SENSES

Have you already mastered mindful breathing? Try adding in the other five senses.

1. Start this exercise with mindful breathing. As you find yourself in a peaceful rhythm, shift your focus.
2. Think about what you feel. Are you lying or sitting? What part of your body is touching the ground or floor? Is it hard or soft? Move your feet/toes or hands/fingers. What do you feel? Once you have explored all the ways that you can touch or feel your surroundings, shift your focus.

3. Think about what you smell. Do you note any aromas? How does this make you feel? Once you have explored this, shift your focus.

4. Think about what you taste. Is it one simple flavor, or can you break it down? How does this make you feel? Once you have explored this, shift your focus.

5. Think about what you hear. Are you inside or outside? What do you hear? Listen closely. Can you identify each individual sound? How do these sounds make you feel? Once you have explored this, shift your focus.

6. Finally, open your eyes. What do you see? Take in all of your surroundings. Look around slowly. Think about how you feel about each item or person you see. Remember to stay in the moment. Bring back your other senses, and use all five senses to make an overall picture of this moment.

7. Now slowly move your focus back to your breathing. Close your eyes, and focus on your breathing. When you feel you are calm and in a peaceful rhythm again, end your practice.

I recommend using one or both of the above exercises for a minimum of a week to see the results. There are many more exercises available out there as well. You can join my blog to find links or simply use a browser search. You can also try other ways on your own. Many use the time during a long run or while exercising to practice mindfulness. Others sit and enjoy nature or listen to relaxing music. Whatever you feel can bring you into the current moment will help you to be more mindful, but remember that the key to building any new habit is consistency and repetition.

Using these exercises or another way to be in the moment and slow life's pace will help you feel relaxed and happy. Mindfulness and relaxation go hand in hand. Once you feel comfortable practicing mindfulness, move on to Chapter 2, where you will learn more about the second pillar of wellness and how relaxation can bring positive changes to your health and wellness.

Chapter 2

RELAXATION FOR THE BODY, MIND, AND SPIRIT

"REMEMBER THAT YOUR MENTAL HEALTH IS A PRIORITY, YOUR INNER PEACE IS ESSENTIAL, AND YOUR SELF-CARE IS A NECESSITY." –UNKNOWN

Now that you have practiced mindfulness, you can move on to Pillar Two of Optimal Wellness—relaxation. If you have not started practicing mindfulness, I suggest you stop and familiarize yourself with mindfulness practices before moving on to relaxation.

What is *relaxation* in terms of wellness? Most people know it is something we do to release tension or become free of stress. But beyond relieving stress and tension, relaxation has many benefits to the human body. When you are relaxed, you will immediately notice a lower heart rate, slower respiratory rate, less anxiety, and decreased sweating. Over time, you may also notice a decrease in blood pressure, better circulation, improved mood, increased metabolism due to lower blood cortisol levels (*cortisol* is a hormone in the body that increases with stress and can have a negative effect on metabolism when at an elevated level), and just feeling better overall.

The "old me" did not know how to relax. When I started treatment after my head injury, a provider asked, "What are your hobbies?"

My reply, "What do you mean?"

She asked again, "What do you do to relax?"

Relax? Really? I said, "I don't have time for hobbies. Before I hit my head, all I did was work and now I just sleep."

I was told it was time for me to learn how to relax, find a hobby, and try to do something for myself. I was seriously at a loss. *What in the world was I supposed to do?* Since my injury, all I ever did was sit around. Isn't that relaxation?

Turns out that sitting around doesn't equate to relaxation. Look at the definition again—release tension or become free of stress. Despite me not being active, I was not relaxing because I was still stressed and anxious. I was not truly taking time for myself or doing things to relieve all of my stress and tension. It was time to get serious about finding a hobby.

FINDING A HOBBY

My neurologist told me doing creative things would help with my brain recovery. My niece took me shopping at the local bookstore, so I could try to find a creative hobby. I could think of nothing! So I tried multiple creative hobbies.

My first attempt at a hobby was origami. Oh, was that a hoot! I was too much of a perfectionist for this and the poor papers were so wrinkled from the folding and refolding that whatever I tried to make ended up a very sad finished product. I know perfectionism is something I should have been working to overcome, but at that point in my life I had yet to discover the art of mindful meditation. (I'm still working on my need for everything to be perfect because I'm still on my journey.)

I tried many other crafty ideas and most ended up in a donation box. About three to four months later, I pulled the crochet needle and yarn back out and tried again. I ended up crocheting my first blanket. It wasn't really the shape of a blanket, but it was kind of square-ish. But to this day, my sister-in-law uses that blanket, and she loves it. This turned into me making five more blankets, then dabbling in other crochet projects. As I improved at this hobby and began enjoying it. I noted that it helped with my migraines when medications weren't offering complete relief. I also noted how I was more relaxed and had fewer headaches.

But the most important point of this is that I'd finally found a way to relax. Crocheting meant I was taking time for myself. I was escaping the stressors in my life, which enabled me to decrease my headaches and relieve anxiety.

From there I searched for more interests that I enjoyed. Now when asked about hobbies, I have a list of different favorite activities. One such hobby is chickens! I absolutely love my chickens and have reveled in the excitement of collecting eggs and watching them when they free range. I also read about them and have gained so much knowledge about chickens, their habits, health concerns and treatments, and so much more. Meeting a friend to walk in the morning, socializing while walking is another activity I have enjoyed. I still crochet and love gifting friends and family with the products of my hobby. I have also enjoyed gardening again. And I've even begun helping my sister-in-law when she makes cakes. I have become pretty good at making animals out of fondant and gum paste.

What's your hobby? Do you have any activities you enjoy, or are your hobbies centered on what everyone else in your life enjoys? Many of us center our lives around family, work, and what life demands of us. When asked about your hobbies, do you answer with something like, "I enjoy spending time with my family" or "I watch my kids play sports"? I am not telling you to ditch the family or kids, but everyone needs quality time for themselves. Mindfulness is important, but spending ten minutes a few times a day being mindful is not enough. You need to find something you love to treat yourself, and for personal development.

There are many ways to relax. You can find a new hobby like crocheting, making origami, walking, running, playing a sport, bird watching, gardening, or raising chickens. You can also do things like just sitting outside taking in the fresh air. Spirituality is another door to relaxation for some individuals. If you are a religious person, finding a church can be very good for you, as fellowship with like-minded people is a very positive activity. Music is also a great option for many. Both listening to and playing music can be very relaxing. Really there are so many options, and the choice is yours! But you must take the first step and make it a priority to discover your passion. Find what allows you to take away the stress and anxiety in your life.

SELF-CARE

In addition to a hobby, don't forget self-care. We often take care of others and forget to take care of ourselves. When was the last time you did something for yourself? You may already schedule self-care for yourself, but if you don't, you need to add it to your routine.

Self-care obviously includes hygiene, but it also can include an occasional spa day, pedicure, or just ensuring you get that nap you need. Meditation can also help with relaxation, as discussed in Pillar One—mindfulness. There are many types of meditation. The meditation types I have practiced are movement, progressive relaxation, and mindfulness (focused) meditation.

We'll discuss different movement meditations in Chapter 7.

Progressive relaxation is a technique where you are talked through relaxation of the body to help relieve anxiety or stress. I was introduced to this type of relaxation years ago by a friend and colleague. She began by having me lay on my back in a comfortable position and talked me through relaxing each individual body part. As I was relaxing that one finger or leg, I was to focus specifically on how that one body part felt. You can find more information on this type of meditation on my website *https://www.hot-mess-to-wellness.com/*. But now that you're familiar with mindfulness, I encourage you to learn about mindfulness meditation.

MINDFULNESS (FOCUSED) MEDITATION

This type of meditation is like mindful breathing, but with practice it can take you deeper into relaxation.

1. Choose a target for your focus. Many will choose to focus on their breath. Some will use an object like a crystal. You can also focus on a sound or other sensation.
2. Find a quiet place and get comfortable. If you are more comfortable sitting, I recommend trying to sit upright, and if on a chair, sit at the edge with both feet on the floor. If you choose to lie down I recommend lying supine (on your back).
3. Close your eyes and clear your mind. Relax your body.
4. Focus on your target. Experience the target, including the sensations you feel. If focusing on your breath, focus on how you feel as you inhale through your nose and exhale through your mouth. If you are focusing on an object, focus on other details such as the other senses of sight, smell, and touch.
5. Calm any internal monologue that strays from the target. If you

think about other things, such as your to-do list, refocus back to your target.

6. Do this for five to ten minutes, refocusing if your mind wanders.

Meditation can be difficult in the beginning. If you find meditation frustrating and notice your mind wandering, just refocus. Don't get upset if you find meditation difficult at first—it can take multiple sessions before you truly feel focused. Begin with brief sessions (about five minutes). If you try one type of meditation and it's not for you, simply try one of the other types of meditation discussed.

If you need more information, you can find articles and audio files where I walk you through multiple types of meditation at *https://www.hot-mess-to-wellness.com/*. This week you should work on ways you can bring relaxation into your life. Write a list and try to work those into your schedule. In Chapter 3, we will discuss Pillar Three—sleep. Bringing mindfulness and relaxation into your life should make sleep easier to tackle.

Chapter 3
RESTFUL SLEEP

"PEOPLE WHO SAY THEY SLEEP LIKE A BABY USUALLY DON'T HAVE ONE." –
LEO J. BURKE

You're doing a great job working on both mindfulness and relaxation to improve your mindset, and to care for not only others but yourself too. We all know that unless you care for yourself, you can't care effectively for others.

I know all too well how easy it is to fall into the habit of caring for others; by focusing outward instead of inward, I let myself suffer. Prior to my injury, I worked long hours and did not focus on my sleep. In this chapter, we will move on to Pillar Three of Optimal Wellness, which involves realizing the effects of having a restful night of sleep.

As a physician I recommend that my patients get eight to ten hours of "restful sleep" every night. The average American gets less than seven hours of sleep a night. But is that restful sleep? It's hard to say because many people don't know what restful truly means. Do you? Don't worry if you don't understand the inner workings of restful sleep because we'll get to know the stages and how they work to refresh your body.

Sleep is a state of decreased responsiveness and metabolism, and it's essential for the body to thrive. You need uninterrupted sleep consisting of all sleep stages for the body to have the time it needs for optimal function. With an appropriate amount of truly restful sleep, you won't feel fatigued or sluggish the next morning. Let's dive into those stages a bit more.

STAGES OF SLEEP

There are five stages of sleep that are divided into one stage of REM (rapid eye movement) and another four stages of non-REM sleep.[2] Let's start with the non-REM, or nREM, stages first.

NON-REM (NREM)

- Stage N1. This is the lightest stage of sleep and occurs as you transition from wakefulness into sleep. This stage is usually less than 10% of an average adult's sleep each night.
- Stage N2. This stage usually follows N1, and you fall into a slightly deeper sleep where you are harder to awaken. This stage is usually around 50% of an average adult's sleep each night.
- Stage N3 & N4. These stages are referred to as "deep sleep," and N4 is a progression from N3 into deeper sleep. These occur usually in the first half of the night. They usually make up around 20 to 25% of an average adult's sleep each night.

During the nREM stages of sleep the body and brain are rested and restored.

REM

- **REM, or rapid eye movement.** This stage is recognized as the time when we dream and when memories are integrated. There are two different phases, and in one of them the eye movement is less frequently noted. During *phasic REM* there are bursts of eye movement, and during *tonic REM*, there's relatively little eye movement. The muscles are less active during tonic REM. It accounts for roughly 20% of the average adult's sleep each night.

All stages of sleep are important and have a part in the body's ability to rest and restore appropriately. Eliminating the time spent in any stage can be detrimental to your wellness. There are many reasons you may not feel rested in the morning when you awake, and the first is likely that you did not have restful sleep. Ask yourself the following questions to assess your sleep habits and efficacy.

1. Do I have a typical bedtime routine?
2. Do I go to bed and wake at roughly the same time every day?
3. Do I have a quiet and dark place to allow my body to sleep restfully?
4. Am I drinking caffeine too late in the day?
5. Am I on a medication that could keep me awake at night?
6. Do I have a known medical condition that awakens me at night?
7. Do I suffer from ADHD, depression, or anxiety?

Carefully consider your answers and be honest with yourself. Many people don't have a bedtime routine, have an inconsistent schedule, and drink caffeine in either a large quantity or too late in the day. Alcohol and tobacco can also have an effect, as well as eating too close to bedtime, especially if you have any issues with acid reflux. Let's take a closer look.

Prior to my injury and when I was working full time, I had multiple detrimental responses to the questions above. I did not have a bedtime routine—I went to bed and awoke at random times (mostly because of my ever-changing work schedule), I drank coffee like a fiend, and I suffered from depression and anxiety, as well as reflux. After my injury this all worsened because I slept too much as a result of the TBI. Now if I note I am having increased fatigue, I go back and ask myself these questions again. This usually helps me to narrow down that my fatigue is likely due to me not getting restful sleep and leads me to a solution resulting in restful sleep again.

BEDTIME ROUTINE

Do you have a bedtime routine? As a pediatrician I ask this question first when chatting with the parents of a child whose complaint is *insomnia* (or inability to fall asleep or stay asleep). Many people want to say yes they have a routine to avoid feeling judged or like they are parenting poorly. You may feel the same way right now. But no judgment here. Our society crams so many activities into our lives that it's very difficult to have the time to wind down before bed.

TV and smartphones are also detrimental to sleep in more than one way. The blue light from these devices is known to decrease the levels of natural melatonin that the body produces, which causes delayed onset of sleep. (More on melatonin later.) Our devices are also quite the distraction and lead us to binge watch Netflix or scroll through social media; in both cases we lose track of time. Before you know it, you're looking at the clock saying, "Oh shit, it's midnight and I have to work in the morning." You rush off to bed and can't fall asleep with all the thoughts running through your mind because you did not take the time to wind down before bed. I'm definitely guilty of all the above!

Let's consider a better way to think about bedtime. What do you enjoy? What calms you? Perhaps you have begun mindful meditation after adopting Pillar One. Maybe you are someone who enjoys journaling. The key to a bedtime routine is that it's supposed to help you wind down and allow your brain to turn off. A routine can be as simple as you want to make it.

One example of a good bedtime routine includes putting down the smartphone and turning off the TV by 8:30 p.m., followed by a shower or bath, completing nightly hygiene (brush teeth, etc.), then journaling for a bit, intending to turn out the lights and go to sleep no later than 10 p.m. Having no screen time two hours before bedtime is recommended, but I am a realist and understand that's difficult.

CONSISTENCY

Whatever routine you decide to adopt, consistency is key. The body has a natural circadian rhythm, which triggers your body to know you must go to sleep. Many people have their body so confused because of their inconsistency. This isn't always their fault.

For instance, consider my old schedule. When I was working prior to my injury, being the Chief of Pediatrics meant I was both running the outpatient pediatric clinic as well as overseeing inpatient medicine. With a team of four military doctors, if I had a shortage of civilian employees, one of us had to cover. Coverage was 24 hours a day if we had admitted patients. There were many night shifts, and a significant share of flipping back and forth between night and day shifts. It was exhausting, and my circadian rhythm didn't know when I was supposed to be sleeping.

You need the same routine every night, even on the weekends. You also need to awaken around the same time *every* morning. This consistency helps your body's circadian rhythm find its way back to normalcy.

PROPER SLEEPING CONDITIONS

Do you fall asleep to music or with the TV playing? As a physician one of my biggest pet peeves is a TV in the bedroom, especially in a child's bedroom. Having noise during sleep can cause accidental arousal and decrease chances of restful sleep. The best environment to sleep in is a cool, completely dark, and quiet room.

Some of you might be thinking, *But my partner snores!* Ear plugs, my friend. My husband has worn them for years. Yes, I am the spouse who used to snore until diagnosed with sleep apnea. And now I have a CPAP machine (more on that later).

CAFFEINE AND OTHER DRUGS

Drugs? You're probably thinking you don't use drugs.

But I would bet you do.

Caffeine, nicotine, prescription medications, vitamins, and alcohol can all be classified as drugs. One of the most widely used drugs, caffeine, often causes sleep issues. We drink so much caffeine in coffee, tea, soda, energy drinks, even water. Yes, I saw flavored water at the store that contains caffeine. We have become an over-caffeinated society, and it's detrimental to our health.

Increased caffeine or caffeine too late in the day can cause sleep disturbances, which then leads to fatigue the next day. Use of caffeine to get through that day also causes our inability to fall asleep the next night, creating a never-ending cycle. The FDA recommends only 400 milligrams (mg) of caffeine daily. Did you know one cup of coffee contains approximately 100 mg of caffeine? This is an 8 ounce cup of coffee, not the 20 ounce travel mug you fill and take to work daily. Think about that. And one shot of espresso has around 60 mg of caffeine! How many shots do you like in your cappuccino?

Most caffeinated sodas contain less at 20 to 30 mg in 8 ounces, but remember many sodas have more than an 8 ounce portion in the bottle or can. Do you drink energy drinks? The average energy drink contains approximately 50 to 70 mg of caffeine per 8 ounces. Be careful thinking these alternatives have less caffeine than coffee because many of those drinks are also more than 8 ounces per can or bottle. Looking at the energy shots, they have around 200mg of caffeine in just one small bottle that you typically ingest all at once. It's quite the eye opener.

Drinking increased amounts of caffeine can have disruptive effects on sleep. Caffeine is a stimulant that can cause trouble when it comes to falling asleep, and that reduces your total sleep time. As a physician I recommend decreasing overall caffeine ingestion, but if that is not feasible, stopping consumption earlier in the day can help.

According to a study in the *Journal of Clinical Sleep Medicine*, you should "refrain from substantial caffeine use for a minimum of 6 hours prior to bedtime."[3] They found people who were consuming caffeine even 6 hours prior to bedtime had loss of sleep. Any loss of sleep that occurs night after night compounds and the effects worsen.

Alcohol can also affect sleep. Yes, alcohol is known as a depressant, and it makes you drowsy and allows you to fall asleep faster. But then it can cause you to awaken before you have the REM stage of sleep. This is a known effect and can worsen if you are a chronic drinker. Less REM sleep causes increased daytime sleepiness the next day. Loss of sleep night after night increases your risk for many disorders and can worsen current disorders.

Nicotine, whether in the form of cigarettes, cigars, a vape, or chewing tobacco, is widely used. I'm not the type of physician that lectures those addicted to nicotine. I would be remiss, however, if I did not mention the effects that nicotine has on sleep. Nicotine is a stimulant. Any nicotine is harmful to the body both in the sleep cycle as well as other processes, which can increase inflammation. Nicotine addiction is definitely hard to overcome, and it's not a primary focus of this book. To me, until you are ready to quit, there is no need to discuss the matter. If you are ready to quit, your medical provider should have multiple ways to help with this. Discuss your choice further with them. Your provider can discuss behavioral methods and medications that can help with nicotine addiction. The US Department of Health and Human Services also has a Smoking Quitline that can help—call 877-44U-QUIT (877-448-7848) for more info.

Prescription medications can also cause sleep disruption. For instance, any of the stimulant ADHD medication taken too late in the day can contribute to issues with falling asleep. Other medications can cause drowsiness, such as allergy medications, so the medical provider advises you to take them before bed. It's very important to know if your medications can influence sleep; discuss this with your medical provider if you're having any abnormal or troublesome effects.

Melatonin is a medication many people equate with better sleep. It's a hormone that regulates the sleep-wake cycle known as your *circadian rhythm*. While melatonin is fairly harmless, it can have side effects and interfere with other medications. Melatonin can be taken in doses up to 10 mg a day, but you should start with a lower dose. It is usually taken thirty minutes before bedtime, but it can be taken up to three hours before bedtime. Many who take it don't understand that taking more than the recommended dose does not necessarily make it more effective. Like any medication, it should be taken in accordance with your provider's recommendation or the instructions on the over-the-counter packaging.

MEDICAL CONDITIONS THAT CAN CAUSE SLEEP DISRUPTIONS

ACID REFLUX

I have suffered from acid reflux for as long as I can remember, and it's a very prevalent diagnosis for many Americans. Obesity and our poor diet are definitely not helping. Beyond possible stomach and chest discomfort (heartburn), acid reflux can also disrupt restful sleep.

If you have this disorder, you should follow these reflux precautions:

- eat smaller meals multiple times daily to ease pressure of the esophageal sphincter
- eat slowly
- avoid fatty, fried, spicy, and acidic foods
- avoid caffeine, alcohol, and nicotine
- stay upright after meals
- eat your last meal at least three hours before bedtime to avoid reflux disruptions to the sleep cycle

Heeding these warnings can reduce your reflux occurrence and hopefully make for more pleasant and refreshing sleep.

INSOMNIA

Insomnia is also a growing diagnosis. *Insomnia* can be both trouble falling asleep and trouble staying asleep, both of which influence your restful sleep.

There are many causes of insomnia including stress/anxiety, some medical conditions, and certain medications. If you're still having issues after following all of the suggestions of this chapter, please visit your medical provider to discuss further evaluation and treatment.

SLEEP APNEA

Sleep apnea affects your breathing while you sleep, and it's a significant disease with a growing impact, likely because of the overall increase in obesity in the US. It can be classified as central or obstructive.

Central sleep apnea means something central (think brain/nervous system) is the cause.

Obstructive sleep apnea occurs when something is obstructing airflow and causing apneic events.

An *apneic event* is when breathing stops for 20 or more seconds. If the oxygen saturation in your tissues (especially your brain) drops to a low level during an apneic episode, it can be especially troublesome. Low levels of oxygen in your tissues means they cannot function, and sustained low levels can kill some tissues.

Sleep apnea is something that can only be diagnosed with polysomnography or a sleep test. Here are some of the symptoms:

- excessive daytime sleepiness
- snoring

- episodes of no breathing, breathing through the mouth, or loud breathing (if you have a bed partner, ask them about this)

You should schedule an appointment with your medical provider if you are experiencing these symptoms.

MAJOR HEALTH CONCERNS CAUSED BY OR WORSENED BY POOR SLEEP

How many times have you had an awful night and gotten little to no sleep? How did you feel the next day? I am guessing it was a rough morning. Your brain was foggy, like it wasn't working well. Some individuals may have felt moody or easily frustrated. Some may have felt easily distracted throughout the day and/or had trouble concentrating. Others may experience physical issues such as fatigue, achiness, or worsening of a chronic medical condition. Let's look into some of these conditions.

COGNITIVE FUNCTION AND MOOD

Poor sleep can cause a decrease in cognitive function, memory, and alertness. And it can decrease productivity. If you had one bad night you can easily repair this with a good night of restful sleep. But if you have night after night of disrupted sleep, this compounds and you cannot just "catch up." Note, as the body ages, the body also takes less time to show effects, and it takes longer to recover from the effects.

You may also notice moodiness after poor sleep. If you don't I'm sure your partner will. Mood changes can also occur with inadequate sleep and worsen as the deficit increases. Inadequate sleep can also worsen your depression and anxiety as well as decrease sex drive. All of these effects connect to the brain not receiving restorative sleep.

ADHD

You may know someone with ADHD, or perhaps you have been diagnosed yourself. *ADHD*, or *attention deficit hyperactivity disorder*, is a disorder in which the brain does not focus well. ADHD can be divided into ADHD with hyperactivity, ADHD with inattentiveness, and ADHD-combined type.

To be diagnosed with ADHD, the patient must show symptoms in two different environments, such as school and home. This enables doctors to ensure we aren't dealing with a behavioral or disciplinary issue. Yet did you know sleep dysfunction can worsen ADHD and sleep disorders can mimic ADHD? When a person gets too little sleep, it causes cognitive functions to decline.

An average person with sleep deprivation can seem as if they have ADHD symptoms. A person with ADHD can also have worsening symptoms of both hyperactivity and inattentiveness if they have poor sleep. Sleep quality should be assessed prior to considering an ADHD diagnosis or any ADHD medication changes.

OTHER DISORDERS

With inadequate sleep also comes increased risk for multiple other diseases and disorders. You may not suffer from these, but if you have a family history or other conditions that predispose you to them, inadequate sleep can increase your risk(s).

The first is a weakened immune system. When the body doesn't get the time it needs for restorative processes, it's like your car not getting its regular maintenance. The immune system can suffer and be weakened. Once the immune system is weakened, other diseases can occur.

Other diseases and disorders that can have increased risk with poor sleep are heart disease, hypertension (elevated blood pressure), and type 2 diabetes. This is not an all-inclusive list, but if you already have these diseases or others, they can worsen without restful sleep. Please follow up with your medical provider with questions about other disorders.

STEPS TO A RESTFUL NIGHT OF SLEEP

Okay, I have thrown a lot of information at you in this chapter. But sleep is very important. To help you achieve a night of restful sleep, here's a recap and some tips. Please do the following things and continue trying them until you can get into a routine.

1. Start a bedtime routine that allows you to turn off screens, relax, and wind down.
2. Avoid blue light exposure (smartphone/TV) for 2 hours prior to bedtime.
3. Try to go to bed and wake up at about the same time every day, even on weekends.
4. Prepare your sleeping quarters—dark, cool, and quiet (wear ear plugs if you need them).
5. Stop all caffeine and nicotine 6 hours prior to your bedtime.
6. Review all side effects of the medications you are taking, and if any cause sleep disturbance, discuss that with your medical provider.
7. Stop eating at least 3 hours prior to bedtime.

8. Don't take daytime naps.
9. Follow all of these steps for a week and see how they help your sleep. Consistency is key.

Now that you've worked on habits to improve sleep, you should start to feel more rested. Next you'll learn the importance of hydration. Water is the single most important nutrient you put into your body. When you are ready to dive in (pun intended), move on to Chapter 4.

Chapter 4
HYDRATION

"Pure water is the world's first and foremost medicine." -
Slovakian Proverb

You are doing great. You are practicing mindfulness, considering the ways you can relieve life's stresses through relaxation, and incorporating a bedtime routine to get the restful sleep you deserve. While you don't need to master each, I recommend attempting to work each pillar into your routine as you read so you are not overwhelmed making multiple changes all at once. Once you feel confident with the first three pillars, move on to Pillar Four of Optimal Wellness—hydration.

"Drink water" is something everyone in any branch of the military has heard! We used to have to carry around two canteens when out in the "field" on a training exercise. There were even times we had to prove we drank water by holding the canteen upside down over our head in formation. Hopefully you were actually drinking that water, otherwise you were soaked. Now things are a little different, but the premise remains—drinking water is imperative to the success of the mission.

I can honestly say that physicians are the worst about hydrating. I was and am still chronically dehydrated. I know, I know, I am writing a book with Pillar Four being about hydration, telling you I am an expert and to drink water, but then I tell you I am chronically dehydrated. What gives?

Well, I'll remind you that I'm on this journey with you, and we all have things we need to work on. Hydration is something I continue to work on.

WHY IS HYDRATION SO IMPORTANT?

The human body can survive up to two months without food, but it can only survive three to five days without water. These are estimates and many other factors can play a role, but this shows the importance of water. Your body is about 70% water, and each cell in your body is roughly 40 to 50% water. Water is an essential part of life.

You've probably heard that people should drink about 8 glasses of water a day, but that's not exactly accurate. Depending on your weight, you should probably drink more. You should drink a minimum of a ½ ounce of water per pound you weigh. For example, if you weigh 150 pounds, drink a minimum of 75 ounces of water a day. For those of you outside America, that would equal out to approximately 2.25 Liters for a person weighing approximately 68 kg (or approximately 33 ml per kg).

The body needs water, but what happens if the body gets too little water? The human body relies on water not only as part of its cell makeup but also for many of the physiologic functions.

Physio what? *Physiologic functions*, the normal functions of the living human body, need hydration and 75% of Americans are chronically dehydrated. There's definitely room for improvement!

EFFECTS OF CHRONIC DEHYDRATION ON THE HUMAN BODY

Water provides structure to the body's cells and is used in every cellular process. Mitochondrial processes that make energy for your cells also use water. Chronic dehydration can cause a decrease in the amount of fluid in cells and throughout the circulatory system. It can also cause increased frequency or intensity of headaches, constipation, and increased risk for urinary tract issues.

Dehydration is also known to cause hypotension (low blood pressure), especially when someone stands quickly (known as *orthostatic hypotension*). You can also suffer from light-headedness and dizziness. The body pulls fluids to various parts for processes critical to survival; an example is when blood vessels sustain an adequate blood pressure by directing fluids centrally from extremities and less important organs when needed. If you're dehydrated, the body cannot perform all of its functions. Other processes will be placed on the back burner, and toxins will not be effectively discarded. You will also age more quickly and have many impaired body functions.

The brain is over 70% water. Without adequate hydration, you may notice impaired cognitive function such as lack of focus, poor memory, or fogginess. You may also have an increased number of headaches or notice more severe headaches.

Water is also critical in the digestive system. Saliva, which is made of water, moistens food and contains the enzymes that begin digestion as you chew. In the stomach, water helps promote the continued digestive process. It's also a component in the stomach's mucus lining, protecting it from its highly acidic environment. Water is also a part of the secretions in the small intestine that include the digestive enzymes doing most of the digestive processes.

Most importantly, however, water is *critically* important in the large intestine (colon). We need adequate amounts of both water and fiber in order for our body to have regular bowel movements. Without adequate hydration, you may suffer from ailments such as dry mouth, halitosis (bad breath), acid reflux, constipation, or abdominal pain.

The urinary tract removes waste, toxins, and extra water from the body. Water helps to transport nutrients to cells, and waste from cells out of the body. If you are chronically dehydrated, you may notice dark urine, decreased urine output, an increase in urinary tract infections, or even kidney stones. When the waste being filtered out does not have enough water to be dissolved, it can precipitate out, increasing your risk of kidney stones.

ADEQUATE HYDRATION

As I discussed earlier you should drink at least half of your weight in ounces of water daily. At my heaviest, I weighed 187 pounds. I should have been drinking a minimum of 94 ounces of water daily. I was not.

I was also suffering from IBS with chronic constipation, having migraine headaches that may have been worsened by my hydration status (or not), having balance issues that may have been worsened by my hydration status (or not). I had a chronically low blood pressure, though, too. At one point, I had a blood pressure of 85/58 at one of my visits to the doctor. My nurse was worried. I wasn't bothered because my normal was around 90/60. Now that I am drinking more water, my blood pressure is in a more normal range of around 120/70.

Could my low blood pressure have been contributing to my

dizziness and balance issues? Absolutely. There is really no way to know, but I am definitely feeling better now, and that's thanks to being more diligent about increasing my water intake.

Drinking 94 ounces of water in a day seems like a bit of a feat, and I would like to share a few tips to make this less daunting. First, you need to be drinking water. You cannot substitute soda, juice, etc. If you are substituting something like soda or juice, you will take in large amounts of added sugar. This is just adding empty calories and not helping with hydration. If you are an athlete doing increased workout sessions or long runs, you may need added sugar and electrolytes, but the average person doesn't need these.

You may say, "But I don't like water." There are ways to make water tasty. You can add natural flavor by using an *infuser*, which is a bottle where you fill an inner compartment with a fruit or vegetable for a hint of flavoring. You can also just place a handful of berries, or a slice of lemon, orange, or cucumber in your glass of water.

Decaffeinated green tea is another drink you can add for hydration. Caffeine is a natural diuretic and causes you to lose more water in the urine, so decaffeinated is a better choice. Green tea has more antioxidants and can help increase the metabolism, as well. It's the better choice for hydration when looking at the forms of tea.

Hydrating throughout the day is crucial. The best time to start your hydration is first thing in the morning. I recommend drinking at least one glass of water first thing before you have anything else. This should be cold water, and adding lemon is beneficial. Drinking a cold glass of water with lemon first thing in the morning can help jumpstart your metabolism. Do this before you get that morning cup of coffee. And as for coffee, it's okay in moderation, but don't include it in the 94 ounces because it doesn't hydrate, especially when caffeinated. Like tea, coffee is a diuretic and causes increased fluid loss in the urine.

When thinking about drinking 94 ounces a day, it seems like an enormous amount of fluid. But break it down. This would be just under 12 (8 ounce) glasses a day or 8 (12 ounce) glasses a day. You can easily do this, but you need a plan because it's easy to get halfway through your day and realize you have forgotten to drink and are behind. Chugging water at the end of the day to make up what you missed will just lead to the kidneys filtering water out so quickly that your body gets no benefit and you end up in the bathroom a lot. Also remember to follow your thirst cues.

If you are chronically dehydrated, you may not feel thirsty until you get yourself into a new routine. Do you feel hungry? Are you really hungry, or are you thirsty? Sometimes thirst can masquerade as hunger. Try drinking some water before eating or even drink some water with a small healthy snack instead of binging on a large amount of food.

Here's an example hydration plan to get adequate amounts throughout the day:

- 16 oz first thing in the morning, flavored with lemon
- 12 oz midmorning with a small healthy snack
- 24 oz with lunch
- 12 oz midafternoon with a small healthy snack
- 24 oz with dinner
- 8 oz just before bed

If you weigh less, you can decrease the ounces to fit your hydration needs. You also may not be able to drink right before bed and that's okay. Change this plan to fit your lifestyle. This is just one example, and it's what I try to stick to. You can also start drinking a glass or bottle of water during a meal or snack, finishing it throughout the rest of the morning or afternoon.

I do want to recommend that most water intake be with a meal or snack because it will help your body to use the water more effectively.

CAN I DRINK TOO MUCH WATER?

There is a condition called *hyponatremia* where the bloodstream has too little sodium. This can be caused by overhydration and usually occurs in athletes or soldiers who are overhydrating with massive amounts of water taken in during a short period of time.

To avoid this issue, focus on attempting to drink half your body weight in ounces, drinking water throughout the day and with other intake such as a meal, or snack. Adding a form of electrolytes like a low-sugar sports drink will help you avoid overhydration, but is usually not necessary unless you have an intense exercise routine causing increased sweating. One way to keep an eye on hydration status is by the color of your urine. Many think clear urine is the goal. It's not. Your urine should be a very light/pale yellow.

- Dark straw-colored urine indicates dehydration and your need for adequate hydration.
- Clear urine indicates overhydration and is likely due to drinking too much water in a short window of time.

Do not be concerned that clear urine is a health risk. If you're not experiencing other symptoms, you should be able to change intake of water, spreading it throughout the day and ensuring that you have other intake to adequately absorb some of the water into the body's cells.

HYDRATION CHECKLIST

Here's a quick checklist for building an effective hydration plan.

1. Drink ½ of your body weight (pounds) in ounces.
2. Fill a water bottle and keep it with you, especially to drink with meals and snacks. Drink through a straw because for whatever reason, we seem to get more fluid intake when using a straw.
3. Drink *water*! (Juice, sports drinks, and soda are full of empty calories/caffeinated coffee and tea dehydrate.).
4. Flavor your water with a small amount of fruit (berries, a slice of lemon or orange) or vegetable (a slice of cucumber). This is just floating, not blended or juiced.
5. Drink decaffeinated green tea, which can be nourishing and hydrating.
6. Start your hydration first thing in the morning.
7. Try to hydrate at mealtime to get the most out of your water.
8. Remember that if you note hunger it may actually be thirst.

These tips can help you to slowly work up to your hydration goal and build a daily habit. If you have trouble getting adequate amounts of fluids in, keep working at it. We all have setbacks on our journey. Brush it off and keep pushing on! If you're an athlete, please discuss hydration further with your coach or trainer because you'll likely need to add an electrolyte replacement.

Now that you have worked on hydration, we need to discuss what you are eating. This is also a very important part of your health and wellness. In Chapter 5, we will begin discussing Pillar Five—healthy eating.

Chapter 5

DITCHING THE DIET

"TO KEEP THE BODY IN GOOD HEALTH IS OUR DUTY, OTHERWISE WE WILL
NOT BE ABLE TO KEEP OUR MIND STRONG AND CLEAR." –BUDDHA

Before we move on to Pillar Five, did you calculate your average daily water needs? How did you keep up with your hydration? You should try to work on hydration for a week to establish the new habit of drinking more. Focusing on one pillar at a time is key. But if you are ready to move on, let's learn about the foods you should be eating and why.

Grubhub, DoorDash, Uber Eats, Postmates, We Deliver—I had all of these apps on my phone when I was homebound shortly after my injury. I sat alone in the dark to keep the migraines from worsening. I felt alone, defeated, overwhelmed. Luckily I had an amazing sister-in-law who saw my struggle and gave me the motivation to keep going.

My provider referred me to the TBI and pain clinics, and with a great medical team I started to improve. I was still struggling with loss of my identity going from the constantly on-the-go, energetic, talkative physician to this blob on the couch. I gained nearly thirty pounds and crossed the threshold to obesity, joining the 40% of Americans that fall into this category.[4]

Of course, I denied my part in the situation. I blamed it on a new medication I was taking and the fact that I could not exercise. Along with obesity came shame, worsening depression, increased exhaustion, and many other issues. As a physician I knew the right answer was to be more active and eat healthy foods. But as a patient at my lowest point I lacked the motivation to do those things.

I began moving more with the help of my adaptive reconditioning program through the Army's Warrior Transition Unit but was still having dizziness and daily migraines. At that point there was no improvement in my diet. I was not getting the results I wanted, so I browsed online and went to the bookstore to search for books that would help me. All I could find were fad diets and books about exercises I couldn't do.

Then I decided I would pave my own way. I knew I needed to eat healthy, but I wanted a plan. I decided to create my own. The next morning was the day I stepped on the scale and saw that horrible number—187! *How can I possibly weigh 187 pounds?*

I began journaling and four pages later I decided this plan needed to be more. Because I had trouble finding a simple plan for the average person, I thought I could write this for myself and share with others. I began writing this book and throughout the process it has held me accountable as well. Throughout this journey, I have learned consistency is key. If I make a mistake I just start from where I left off and keep moving forward.

WHAT IS HEALTHY EATING?

First things first, throw out the food pyramid and low-fat mantra. That was one of the biggest mistakes this nation made. Now we look at the MyPlate diet and I partially incorporate this, but there is so much more to knowing what to put on your plate.

The bottom line is that you don't need a fancy "diet plan"—that means no paleo, Atkins, keto, etc. You don't need to cut out all carbohydrates because certain carbohydrates have some nutrients your body needs. In fact, you should never completely cut anything out of your diet, especially if you are the type of person who knows you will later end up binging.

Yet there are certain foods you need to cut back on because our bodies were not made to consume them in excess. You also need to pay attention to portion sizes and labels. The American diet comprises large portion sizes that are sometimes two or more actual serving sizes. This is a huge part of obesity, along with many people thinking they are eating a "healthy" food that is really not all that good for them. The rules of advertising aren't strict, and if you take the time to read the ingredients on a food you'll see that it has ingredients that will instead cause weight gain and increased inflammation in the body. We will discuss all of these separately.

PORTION SIZES VERSUS SERVING SIZES

Portion sizes are incredibly oversized in America, and this trend is spreading across the globe. A key part to eating healthy is knowing the proper serving size, or in other words, ensuring you're eating the recommended amount.

Wait a minute. Serving size? Portion size? What is the difference?

The *portion size* is the amount of food you "portion" out onto your plate and eat. The *serving size* is a standardized measurement that's used to quantify the recommended amount of the food you are eating; it's listed on the labels of all packaged food.

Using the MyPlate food groups, standardized measurements give the recommended serving size of each subgroup of food.[5] For instance, did you know the recommended serving size for a steak is 3 ounces? The next time you go to the steak restaurant, look at the menu again. Most of the steaks on the menu are 8, 12, sometimes even 20 or 24 ounces. This is just one example of the large portions we eat in America.

ESTIMATING PORTION SIZES

The best way to measure portion sizes is to avoid overestimating and stay close to the recommended serving size. Using a measuring cup/ spoon or kitchen scale can aid in these measurements. Most of us don't carry around a measuring cup though. The good news is that there are other simple comparisons you can use.

- Fruit - The recommended serving size is ½ cup chopped or a medium-sized whole piece of fresh fruit (about the size of a tennis ball). If eating dried fruit, the serving size is ¼ cup.
- Vegetables - The recommended serving size is ½ cup cooked (again think tennis ball) and 1 cup if raw (2 tennis balls).
- Starches (rice, pasta, potatoes, bread) - The recommended serving size is ½ cup (think tennis ball), or 1 piece of bread or tortilla and only ½ of a bagel or burger bun.
- Meat (beef, chicken, fish) - The recommended serving size is 3 oz or about the size of your palm or a deck of cards.
- Other forms of protein (beans, nuts, peanut butter) - The recommended serving size is ½ cup of beans (think tennis ball) or 2 Tablespoons of nuts or peanut butter (about the size of a ping-pong ball).
- Fats (oils, dressings) - The recommended serving size is 1 Tablespoon (about half the size of a ping-pong ball).

- Dairy - The recommended serving size for milk is 1 cup (8 oz), and cheese is 1 ounce (about the size of four dice).

Using the above recommended serving sizes and measuring all of your food initially will empower you with info on true serving sizes. Once you get the hang of it, you won't need to measure. Sometimes you will eat more than one serving in a sitting, and that's okay. Eating a 20-ounce steak when a typical serving size is 3 ounces (and you should only be eating 2 to 3 servings of meat a day), is not okay.

Now you know. Knowledge is power.

WHAT SHOULD I BE EATING?

The average meal consists of large portions of meat, starch, and sometimes a vegetable. Let's think of a visit to the local steakhouse for a meal. After being seated, a basket of bread appears. You eat one roll and promise yourself you are only eating one. You order and that wonderful appetizer arrives. You enjoy a bite of cheese sticks, calamari, chips and cheesy artichoke dip, fried mushrooms, etc. Then your salad arrives. You asked for dressing on the side and only use half. You are very proud you did not overindulge. You finish your salad, and shortly after your meal arrives. Oh, that steak looks wonderful. You ordered the 8-ounce sirloin with sautéed mushrooms and mashed potatoes. That was delicious. Dessert? Maybe not tonight. Okay, let's look at the meal you just ate.

- Meat - 8 oz (2 and ⅔ servings)
- Starch - 1 roll, 2 servings potatoes (there was at least 1 cup on the plate), breading, or chips in the appetizer (3 to 4 servings)
- Vegetable - salad, sautéed mushrooms (1 to 1 ½ servings)

- Fruit - 0 servings
- Other fats
- Maybe a little dairy if you had cheese sticks or cheesy artichoke dip

When you look at it that way it doesn't seem so healthy, does it? The diet should consist of more vegetables and fruit, and less starch and meat. MyPlate is divided into four sections of grains (starch), vegetables, fruits and protein, accompanied by a smaller circle representing dairy. This is the USDA guidance, but many studies since the MyPlate was established have shown that an even larger increase in vegetables is beneficial. My recommendations would be:

- Vegetables - 7-8 servings daily
- Fruit - 2-3 servings daily
- Meat – 2-3 servings daily (remember a serving is 3 ounces)
- Grain - 2 servings daily
- Dairy - 2 servings daily
- Nuts and Legumes - 1 serving daily
- Fats and Oils - 2 servings daily
- Sweets and Added Sugars - 2-3 servings a week (do not eat daily)

Now let's say you know the correct serving sizes and how to portion your food, but you go out to eat and think you have to eat everything on the plate because you spent hard-earned money and don't want to be wasteful.

Or maybe you buy that healthy granola bar and are so proud that you are eating right. Did you read the label?

Perhaps you buy a package of nuts thinking you are going to snack on them instead of chips. You sit down on the couch and dig in. You end up eating the whole bag. Healthy choice, right?

Unfortunately, these are all examples of what not to do.

DO YOU REALLY KNOW WHAT IS IN YOUR FOOD?

Thinking about the granola bar, do you still think it was a healthy choice? No, it wasn't. Why is that? Many granola bars contain hidden sugars, chemicals, and fats that we do not need and additives to keep them fresh. That's why label reading is very important.

When learning to read a label, you need to first note the serving size and how many serving sizes are present in the package. Sometimes you may be taking in double or triple what you thought because you did not look to see you were eating two or three servings.

Also, make sure you are reading the label ingredients. Can you pronounce all the ingredients? Fresh whole foods have names we can pronounce unlike many of the synthetic ingredients found in processed food; they're added to give food a longer shelf life.

If you cannot pronounce it, the ingredient is likely not something you want to put into your body, however if you question whether an ingredient is healthy you can easily look it up. Some words sound harmful and are actually just the opposite. For example, the chemical name for water is H_2O or dihydrogen oxide. This sounds like a chemical we shouldn't ingest when it's just plain old water.

Another way to know what you are eating is to eat whole foods like fresh fruits and vegetables and home-cooked, fresh meals. If you cook the meal yourself, you know the ingredients used to make the meal. You can go even further and raise your own produce, and in some cases even animals.

After the pandemic shutdown, backyard chicken flocks increased exponentially. I have my own flock but not because of the state of the world. I was raised a country girl and have wanted them for many years. My flock produces high quality eggs that I know are not chemically treated in any way. I also have a small garden. If you cannot plant a garden or raise your own meat or eggs, another healthy choice is buying locally. I try to buy all the meat I cook in meals from a local source. The meat I buy is organic and grass-fed beef. Organic and grass-fed beef is the healthiest choice, but many times is also the most expensive. And any produce I use in addition to what I raise is also bought locally. Buying locally, you have a better idea of how your food was raised. Shopping locally is also better for the environment because it decreases transport of product cross-country.

WAYS TO AVOID UNHEALTHY EATING TRAPS

Here are a few ways you can avoid unhealthy eating traps.

- **Read labels.** Reading the label on the food you eat is important. Nutrition facts can help you know the appropriate serving size. Some products have two or more servings, and you think you are taking in a smaller number of calories than you consume. The label also lists ingredients from the highest percentage of product to the lowest. The product will mostly be made of the first few ingredients.

- **Portion your food.** Make sure you portion food onto a plate rather than eating from the package. This will help you eat the correct serving size and not overindulge. It's also beneficial to use the correct tools when you are measuring your portion sizes. Use measuring cups and spoons or a kitchen scale. Once you are comfortable estimating portion sizes at the correct serving size, you can stop measuring. It is helpful to spot check now and then to make sure you are still estimating correctly.

- **Stop getting up-sized meals.** The temptation to get that large meal for an extra $0.49 is sometimes hard to avoid, but adding the extra food is increasing your portion size well above the recommended serving size. If you are eating in a restaurant and the food will can be stored for later consumption, ask for a to-go container at the beginning of the meal so you can stow away any food above the recommended serving size. That can lower the temptation to overindulge.

- **Sit down to eat and do not eat on the go.** You will likely eat unhealthy choices if eating on the go, and you tend to eat more. Rushing through a meal can also lead you to eat more. People who take the time to sit and eat slowly and drink water with their meal will eat less.

Now that you have the basic principles, let's discuss the different food types. In Chapter 6, we will continue discussing Pillar Five and delve into what foods are healthy and what to avoid.

Chapter 6

WHAT FOODS ARE HEALTHY?

"YOUR DIET IS A BANK ACCOUNT. GOOD FOOD CHOICES ARE GOOD INVESTMENTS." -BETHENNY FRANKEL

When I was at my lowest point post-injury, I was not eating the right foods. I didn't care what I was eating because I was looking for comfort in my favorites—pizza, burgers, starches like mashed potatoes and French fries, and sweets. This led me to gain weight. At the time I had no idea that all of these foods were also likely contributing to my fatigue and increased inflammation. In researching for this book, I realized the increased carbohydrates and sugars can cause increased inflammation. I started trying to eat healthier foods and have made a list of the foods recommended and the foods not recommended.[6]

As we discuss Pillar Five, we need to look into eating healthy. There are foods I recommend because of their health benefits. These are on my Recommended List. Some foods may have risk factors associated with them, but the benefits outweigh any slight risk; they are also on my Recommended List. Other foods on the Recommended List are not necessarily bad for you, but they may have risks associated with them such as causing inflammation if eaten too frequently. Other foods you may be surprised to find I do not recommend. They will obviously be on my Not Recommended List. Keep reading as I look more closely at the different kinds of food we consume.

VEGETABLES

Vegetables are the most important food you eat. You should eat 7 to 8 servings of vegetables a day. You should also eat a variety of vegetables to increase the different nutrients you are consuming. Plants have protein, but much less protein than meat. If you are vegetarian or vegan, please note that you need to look at your protein intake, as well as supplement with Vitamin B_{12} to make sure you do not end up with a deficiency. Plants are also low in iron, calcium, and omega-3 fats. If you aren't receiving these in another way, you'll need supplementation.

Fiber may be the most important reason to ensure you eat enough vegetables and fruits. Plants are high in fiber and to have proper digestion, you need fiber and fluid. Remember our constipation conversation from the hydration chapter? In order to bulk up stool, you need fiber. The average person eats an average of 10 grams of fiber daily. The daily recommended amount of fiber for men is 25 grams daily and women is 35 grams daily. We fall incredibly short in this category. Increasing vegetables in your diet will help increase fiber in your diet, as well as increase other needed nutrients.

Vegetables and fruit also have the nutrients needed to feed the microbes, or bacteria that move digestion along, in our intestines. These microbes comprise our microbiome. The actual definition of a *microbiome* is the microorganisms in an environment. A healthy microbiome in the intestines is very important for wellness.

You may have heard the terms prebiotic and probiotic. *Prebiotics* are the nutrients in the foods we eat and feed the gut bacteria. *Probiotics* are the strains of "good" bacteria that live in the gut and can be introduced by eating a variety of vegetables and fruit, or by taking a supplement. We need these "good" bacteria to have a complete microbiome that can help keep the "bad" bacteria from making us sick.

Eating a higher variety of plants in our diet allows for different prebiotics to be consumed by the bacteria to make sure you have a diverse microbiome. Yet increasing the microbiome and feeding it can cause increased gas if done too quickly or if you are constipated. Make sure you treat constipation first and add the vegetables slowly.

Vegetables come in a variety of colors, shapes, and sizes. Have you ever heard the phrase "eat the rainbow"? That's referring to eating a variety of vegetables and fruits in all the colors of the rainbow. Most vegetables are recommended and eating a larger variety is important. Read below for more.

RECOMMENDED

- Red vegetables – bell pepper, fingerling potatoes, onion, radishes, tomatoes
- Orange vegetables – acorn squash, bell pepper, carrots, pumpkin
- Yellow vegetables – spaghetti squash, squash
- Green vegetables (may be white with green leaves) – arugula, artichoke, asparagus, avocado, bell pepper, bok choy, broccoli, brussels sprouts, cabbage, cauliflower, celery, chili pepper, collard greens, cucumber, escarole, fennel, garlic, kale, kohlrabi, leaf lettuce, leek, mustard greens, okra, onion (white or green), parsnip, romaine lettuce, rutabaga, seaweed, shallots, spinach, tomatillo, turnip greens, watercress, zucchini (green summer

squash)

- Purple vegetables – beets, cabbage (technically red), eggplant, fingerling potatoes, radicchio
- Brown vegetables – Mushrooms, which aren't really a vegetable, but a fungus (cremini, portabella, shiitake)

RECOMMENDED IN MODERATION OR NOT RECOMMENDED

- Button mushrooms – avoid (no nutritional value)
- Iceberg lettuce – avoid (no nutritional value)
- Sweet corn – only 2x weekly (technically a grain)
- Sweet potatoes – only 2x weekly (high starch content)
- White potatoes – avoid unless fingerling potatoes (which contain less starch)

FRUIT

Fruit is the next most important food group, although per the MyPlate diet, I feel we are educated to eat too many servings. Although fruit is important and has fiber and needed nutrients, many fruits have a high amount of sugar. Natural sugar is healthier for you than table or artificial sugar, but too much natural sugar can be detrimental to health, especially in someone suffering from obesity, pre-diabetes, or diabetes.

I recommend 2 to 3 servings daily, and you should choose the fruits that are on the Recommended List. If you are diabetic, please discuss these recommendations further with your medical provider; they will probably recommend only 1 cup daily or even less depending on how well controlled your blood sugar is.

You should eat fruit whole. One thing we see in the pediatric clinic is high juice consumption. Juice unfortunately has poor nutritional value and high sugar content, and it always causes the skinny kid to get skinnier and the obese kid to get heavier. Do not drink fruit juice and think it counts as a fruit serving. When drinking your fruit, you are getting all the sugar and none of the fiber. Even if you are juicing at home, that's not as healthy as eating the whole fruit. The fiber is in the pulp, the most discarded part in the process of juicing.

What about fruit juice in the store? Leave it in the juice aisle. Even the juices advertising 100% pure fruit juice are not healthy. One of my biggest pet peeves as a pediatrician is the consumption of juice instead of drinking water and eating whole fruit. Eat the whole fruit and choose a diverse amount of fruit. Remember to "eat the rainbow," just as we discussed with vegetables.

RECOMMENDED

- Red fruits – cherries, guava, pomegranate, raspberries, strawberries, watermelon
- Orange fruits – apricots, grapefruit, mango, nectarine, orange, papaya, peach, tangerine
- Yellow fruits – lemon, durian (although very stinky), star fruit
- Green fruits (may be white) – kiwi, lime, dragon fruit, lychee
- Blue fruits – blueberries
- Purple fruits – acai berries, blackberries, fig (not dried), plums, pluots

RECOMMENDED IN MODERATION OR NOT RECOMMENDED

- Banana – only 2-3 servings per week (high sugar content)
- Dried fruit – avoid, especially if commercially made (high sugar content)

- Grapes – less than 1 serving daily (very high level of sugar)
- Pineapple – less than 1 serving daily (very high level of sugar)

FISH AND SEAFOOD

Fish and seafood should be a large part of your diet, because they include omega-3 fatty acids, such as DHA, which can decrease your risk for heart disease, improve cognition, and decrease anxiety and depression. But you have to be selective when you are picking out your fish. Farmed fish are now very popular, but they're kept in small areas and fed inappropriate feed. This can cause the fish you buy to not have all the nutrients a wild caught fish contains.

Also, as you have likely heard, fish and other seafood can have elevated levels of mercury. The larger wild caught fish are more likely to have higher levels because they are larger fish. Because of the fear of consuming mercury, many people, especially pregnant women will avoid fish altogether. There is a safe way for you, even if pregnant, to consume fish. Choose smaller wild caught fish such as sardines, herring, and anchovies.

RECOMMENDED

- Wild salmon that is truly wild caught ("Atlantic Salmon" is many times farm raised)
- Small fish (smaller means fewer possible toxins) wild caught
- Shrimp, oysters, clams, mussels, scallops

NOT RECOMMENDED

- Large fish such as swordfish (more likely to contain toxins such

as mercury)
- Fish that are not wild caught (farmed)

MEAT AND POULTRY

Animal muscle is the only human source containing Vitamin B_{12}. It also has Vitamin E, D, other B vitamins, multiple enzymes, essential amino acids, antioxidants, and minerals like zinc and iron. These are already in easily absorbed conformations. Plants contain many of these but not in the same conformations. And the human body has to work harder to convert them into usable nutrients. Meat is most known for the protein it contains and although you can get protein from vegetables, eating a plant-based diet can lead to difficulty getting the daily recommended value.

When choosing meat, make sure you look at the source. Many large-scale operations will keep animals in small areas and feed them unhealthy diets including grains. Small areas where the animals cannot move around cause increased risk for disease and poor health of the animals. This poor health causes the resulting meat to be lower quality and is less likely to contain the nutrients you need.

The best way to know how your meat was raised is to either raise it yourself or buy locally. As many of us cannot raise our own beef, buying locally is the next best choice. Buying from a local farmer not only allows you to know the health of the animal but also supports small locally owned farms. (And it's an environmental bonus if the product doesn't have to travel cross-country.)

Meat – Pasture-raised meat is recommended (increased omega-3 fatty acids and other nutrients), but if you cannot buy this, grain-fed is better than not having any protein and nutrient intake.

RECOMMENDED

- Pasture-raised beef, lamb, or pork
- Venison
- Elk
- Bison
- Organ meat from the above animals (nutrient dense)

RECOMMENDED IN MODERATION (IF NITRITE FREE AND PASTURE-RAISED)

- Bacon
- Ham
- Sausage
- Salami

NOT RECOMMENDED - TRY TO AVOID IF POSSIBLE

- Processed meat
- Hot dogs unless 100% Beef or Pork
- Bacon, Sausage, and Salami (if not nitrite free)

Poultry and eggs - Pasture-raised chicken meat and eggs are recommended (increased omega-3 fatty acids and other nutrients), but if you cannot buy this, grain-fed is better than not having any protein and nutrient intake.

RECOMMENDED

- Pasture-raised chicken, turkey, and duck

- Eggs from pasture-raised chickens, turkeys, and ducks
- **Eat whole eggs instead of egg whites—the yolk is the most nutritious part of the egg!

DAIRY

For adults following the MyPlate diet, dairy products are recommended at every meal. I do not agree with this. The average teen or adult does not need 3 (8 oz) glasses of milk a day, especially for those who have obesity—that much milk will increase caloric intake. Plus, two glasses daily is sufficient for the nutrients needed.

Also, milk is not a good idea for many of you who may be lactose intolerant or have issues such as irritable bowel syndrome (IBS), intolerance to milk protein, or a milk protein allergy. As a child, I am sure you remember all the "Got Milk" commercials. You were also likely given milk for school lunch. We were taught that milk is something we have to drink. While milk contains calcium, Vitamin A, B_6, B_{12} and (added Vitamin D) as well as some fatty acids and minerals. It also has enzymes that can cause an issue with digestion.

We were also taught milk is needed for the growth of strong bones, but increased exercise and movement daily is just as important for you to build strong bones as a child and young adult. There are also more sources for calcium than just milk including spinach, turnip greens, blackstrap molasses, bok choy, almonds, and other sources of dairy such as yogurt and cheese.

Also, milk is now full of hormones and other additives. If drinking milk, you should look for pasture-raised dairy, which is higher in omega-3 fatty acids and lower in the inflammatory omega-6 fatty acids, but if you cannot buy this, milk from grain-fed is better than not having any dairy intake.

RECOMMENDED

- Whole milk from pasture-raised cows or goats (goat milk is less inflammatory for those with intolerance or allergy to milk)
- Butter from pasture-raised cows or goats
- Ghee
- Cheese from pasture-raised cows or goats
- Yogurt from pasture-raised cows or goats with NO added sugar
- Kefir from pasture-raised cows or goats

NOT RECOMMENDED

- Low-fat or fat free milk (fat is not the issue with milk)
- Sugary dairy drinks or chocolate milk
- Yogurt with sugar added
- Processed cheeses

FATS

Fat has been given a bad rap. We were taught they will lead to not only obesity but also heart disease. Yet fat is not the leading cause of heart disease and high cholesterol, which we once believed. The thought that fat caused obesity led to the trend for low-fat diets. Low-fat diets then led to increased carbohydrate consumption, which is what truly contributed to the obesity epidemic. We all ate more processed carbohydrates and replaced animal fats with refined vegetable oils that promoted inflammation and led to increased cholesterol and heart disease. Everything we were told was the opposite of the truth.

Fat is essential for life. The human body needs fat for brain development and growth, to build hormones, for healthy cell membranes, and many more physiologic functions. Fat increases metabolism and does not spike sugar levels. Whereas, sugars and carbohydrates cause spikes in sugar levels which triggers release of both insulin and insulin-like growth factor. The release of this growth factor then causes an increase in growth in fat cells. Fat does not cause this. Fat also helps the body absorb nutrients in other foods. For example, eating a small amount of healthy oil on a salad helps the body absorb the nutrients in the vegetables. It's important to note, though, that the fat we eat needs to be naturally occurring, not refined fats and oils. We also need to remember fat should be consumed in moderation and per the recommendations discussed in the previous chapter.

Omega-3 fatty acids are the most important fat we ingest. Both omega-3 and omega-6 fatty acids are essential fatty acids and are not created in the body. We need to consume these in our diet. You may have heard of DHA. It is one ingredient in baby formula to help with brain growth. DHA is an omega-3 fatty acid. Omega-3 fatty acids reduce inflammation, protect the brain, and promote cardiovascular health. They can be found in flax seeds, walnuts, eggs, fatty fish, and grass-fed meat.

Omega-6 fatty acids can cause inflammation. They are found in nuts and seeds and therefore in the refined oils we are eating. Many people are consuming omega-6 fatty acids without knowing it because of the refined oils used in so many foods. Increased intake of omega-6 fatty acids is not healthy. Balance between omega-3 fatty acids and omega-6 fatty acids is the key.

Americans eat a ratio of 1 omega-3 fatty acids to 10 to 20 omega-6 fatty acids. You should eat more omega-3 fatty acids in a ratio closer to 1:1. Studies show, a diet high in omega-6 fatty acids and low in omega-3 fatty acids can increase inflammation, while a diet that includes balanced amounts of each can reduce inflammation. One study in particular done by The Center for Genetics, Nutrition and Health showed that "high omega-6 fatty acid intake and a high omega-6/omega-3 ratio are associated with weight gain" as well as increased insulin resistance.[7]

RECOMMENDED

- Extra virgin olive oil (do not cook at high temperature)
- Ghee, great for cooking (high smoke point)
- Lard or tallow if from pasture-raised animal
- Butter from pasture-raised cows or goats
- Coconut oil

NOT RECOMMENDED

- All processed and hydrogenated oils
- Margarine
- Shortening
- Sunflower, corn, soybean, and cottonseed oils contain large amount of omega-6 fatty acids

BEANS

Beans, also known as legumes, are thought to have a high amount of protein. They do have protein, but not as much as you would get in meat; they also have different amino acids than meat. The amino acids in legumes are not as beneficial in building muscle as those found in meat.

Beans do have the advantage of containing fiber, but they're also full of carbohydrates. They have many other nutrients as well and are inexpensive. Note that if you suffer from pre-diabetes or diabetes, you should not consume beans regularly. If you do not suffer from these conditions, beans can be part of a healthy diet. However, the saying "beans, beans the magical fruit" is also something to keep in mind. Beans promote the overgrowth of bacteria in the intestine, causing increased gas and can cause systemic inflammation in some people.

RECOMMENDED

- Green beans (very low in starch)
- Snow peas or green peas (very low in starch)
- Lentils
- Black beans
- Garbanzo beans
- Black-eyed peas
- Edamame (men of child-bearing age should not eat soy products because it can lower sperm count)
- Soybean based foods like tofu or tempeh (men of child-bearing age should not eat soy products because it can lower sperm count)
- Mung beans
- Fava beans (unless individual has a known or possible G6PD deficiency)

NOT RECOMMENDED - THE FOLLOWING ARE TOO HIGH IN STARCH (CARBOHYDRATES)

- Kidney beans

- Baked beans
- Lima beans
- Peanuts (high in omega-6 fatty acids and toxins that can cause allergic reactions)
- Peanut butter (also full of sugars)

NUTS

Nuts, like fats, are not bad for you. You should eat a handful of nuts daily to lower your risk for cardiovascular disease and heart attack. Eating nuts can also increase your metabolism and decrease abdominal fat. Certain nuts have increased health benefits. See the chart below, which includes data on health benefits including the nuts with increased levels of antioxidants, omega-3 fatty acids, and other minerals and vitamins. I tried to rank them, but there are so many significant benefits in all of these. Explore the benefits listed and choose based on what you like and what would benefit you most. I recommend a handful of a mixture of the following nuts every day.

Nut	Benefits
Almonds	Can lower bad cholesterol Can lower risk of cardiovascular disease Contain cancer fighting antioxidants Can increase growth of beneficial bacteria in the intestines Contain Vitamin E, magnesium, and ~3.5 grams of fiber per handful

Nut	Benefits
Pistachios	Can improve arterial function and blood flow May help reduce the rise in blood sugar after a meal Contain ~3 grams of fiber per handful
Walnuts	Can lower bad and total and raise good cholesterol Can lower risk of cardiovascular disease Can reduce inflammation, improving multiple chronic diseases Can improve arterial function and blood flow Contain magnesium, and ~2 grams of fiber per handful
Cashews	Can improve metabolic syndrome (decrease bad cholesterol or lower blood pressure) Contain magnesium, and ~1 gram of fiber per handful
Pecans	Can lower bad cholesterol and triglyceride levels Contain cancer fighting antioxidants Contain manganese and copper and ~2.5 grams of fiber per handful
Macadamia nuts	Can lower bad and total cholesterol Can lower risk of cardiovascular disease Can reduce inflammation, improving multiple chronic diseases Contain cancer fighting antioxidants Contain ~2.5 grams of fiber per handful

Nut	Benefits
Brazil nuts	Can lower bad cholesterol Can lower risk of cardiovascular disease Can reduce inflammation, improving multiple chronic diseases Contain cancer fighting antioxidants Contain high levels of selenium (aids in digestion, metabolism, thyroid function) Contain magnesium, and ~2 grams of fiber per handful
Hazelnuts	Can lower bad and total cholesterol, as well as triglycerides Can reduce inflammation, improving multiple chronic diseases Contain cancer fighting antioxidants Can improve arterial function and blood flow Contain Vitamin E, magnesium, and ~3.5 grams of fiber per handful

NOT RECOMMENDED

- Nuts covered in sugar or chocolate
- Nut butters (because of the added oil and sugars), eat in moderation if made at home or pure

SEEDS

Seeds, like nuts, can have many health benefits too. Many contain similar nutrients. Flax seeds contain omega-3 fatty acids, helping prevent and treat constipation. Sesame seeds are a great source of protein. Seeds can be added to many different foods such as salads or smoothies.

RECOMMENDED

- Pumpkin seeds
- Chia seeds
- Flax seeds
- Sesame seeds

NOT RECOMMENDED

- Refined oils made from seeds (flax or sesame in small amounts are okay)

GRAINS (STARCHES)

Did you know grains were not consumed by our ancestors? Grains are the seeds of grasses and did not even exist as a food group until industrial farming. If eating a true whole grain, though, it can be healthy. Unfortunately many whole grain foods aren't really whole grain.

Whole wheat bread is usually made from wheat flour instead of whole grains, and as a result it's not as healthy as labeling advertises it to be. Wheat flour is ground-up grain, and the fiber that makes whole grains healthy is now broken down and has no benefit to your body. In that form it's just starch, which is essentially a more complex form of sugar. Wheat flour is not really any healthier than white flour. Using a flour made from almonds or coconuts is a healthier choice. Diabetics should not be eating increased amounts of grains because they are pure starch, and a diabetic should only consume 25 to 50 grams of starch daily.

One of the current trends in America is removing gluten from the diet. While gluten can cause issues, most people do not have a gluten allergy. Another pet peeve of mine is the gluten-free craze. Many people do not understand the difference between gluten sensitivity, celiac disease, and a true wheat allergy. There is no allergy to actual gluten.

The only people who need to avoid gluten indefinitely are those with celiac disease, which is a form of irritable bowel disease (not to be confused with irritable bowel syndrome). Celiac disease is an autoimmune disease that can develop at any age and is manifested when an individual eats gluten. With consumption of gluten, the body responds by attacking the small intestine, causing damage and decreased absorption. Symptoms include severe abdominal pain, chronic diarrhea, vomiting, anemia (iron deficiency), failure to thrive, unwanted weight loss, or fatigue. If you are suffering from multiple symptoms listed, this could be celiac disease or one of many other disorders including constipation. If you have questions, you need to contact your medical provider. This can only be diagnosed with blood testing or an endoscopic procedure.

HOW DO I KNOW IF I SHOULD AVOID GLUTEN?

There are really four types of people when it comes to gluten: those with celiac disease, those with true gluten sensitivity, wheat allergy (rare), and those that have none of the above. If you are diagnosed with celiac disease, avoid *all* gluten. If you have a true wheat allergy, obviously you should also avoid wheat. An allergy is very rare and will manifest symptoms as any allergy would to include hives, anaphylaxis (swelling of throat or trouble breathing), or swelling of the lips or face.

If you have a sensitivity, you may notice increased gas and bloating or change in bowel habits. You can restrict your diet to see if there is an improvement in your symptoms. As with any food, a sensitivity does not necessarily mean a complete restriction of that food for the rest of your life. If you have a food sensitivity and not a true allergy, you can completely remove it from your diet, but sometimes that can be more detrimental because of the nutrients you will also be restricting. Slowly adding the food back into your diet can be achieved if done properly. If you have any question of whether it is a sensitivity or allergy, consult your medical provider.

If you do not belong in the above categories, there is no reason for you to restrict gluten from your diet, especially since grains should not be a major portion of a healthy diet.

RECOMMENDED

- The following list are the most nutritious grains and any not listed should be eaten less frequently:
- Rye (whole-kernel)
- Amaranth
- Millett
- Quinoa
- Wheat bran (outside covering of the seed that has increased fiber)

NOT RECOMMENDED

- Any refined grains

BEVERAGES

Beverages, especially those with sugar or artificial sweetener, are one of the primary culprits of hidden calories.

RECOMMENDED

- Water, water, water! - filtered if possible
- Decaffeinated fresh brewed tea, green tea is preferred (no sugar)
- Caffeinated fresh brewed tea in moderation, green tea is preferred (no sugar)
- Decaffeinated coffee
- Caffeinated coffee in moderation (only 16 oz daily)
- Wine in moderation (only 1 serving - 5 oz daily)
- Liquor in moderation (only 1 serving - 1 oz daily and do not mix with sugar filled drink)
- Coconut water (read the label and look for low or no sugar)

NOT RECOMMENDED

- Anything containing added sugars
- Enhanced waters such as Vitamin water or sports drink–sponsored waters
- Any smoothies or fresh juices you did not make yourself (many contain hidden sugars)
- Drink any fresh squeezed juice you make yourself in moderation (fresh fruit is healthier)
- Beer (made from grains, increasing calories)

SWEETENERS

Sugar is a mainstay in the diet. It is included in many things from baked goods to drinks. I live in the South and sweet tea is a staple down here. Sugar has been shown to increase inflammation. It is not a healthy food and is actually on the Not Recommended List. Below are some substitutions that are better for you.

RECOMMENDED

- Monk fruit
- Stevia products
- Coconut sugar
- Molasses
- Pure maple syrup
- Pure local honey

NOT RECOMMENDED

- Anything not listed as recommended or sweeteners that you may see on a food label that cannot be easily pronounced

If you are reading this book, you likely need to increase the recommended foods and decrease the foods not recommended. Now that you know what you should eat, you can start working toward adding the different types of recommended foods into your diet.

Remember that no one is perfect, and I understand how hard it is to stop eating the Not Recommended foods. I have a very hard time with this too. Have you heard the saying that you should eat to live and not live to eat? Well, I live to eat. This part of my journey will be a lifelong journey for me.

Take some time to work on adding foods from the Recommended List before moving on. Use the ideas above and I have also made a nitty gritty cheat sheet you can print to help you stay on track. Visit *https://www.hot-mess-to-wellness.com/copy-of-resources* to sign up for my community and download your free copy. Once you are ready to move on, we can talk about getting you into motion.

Chapter 7
LET'S GET MOVING

"IT DOES NOT MATTER HOW SLOWLY YOU GO AS LONG AS YOU DO NOT STOP." —CONFUCIUS

We are nearing the end of this guide. At this point, we have discussed five of the Seven Pillars. Remember this is a gradual habit-building process. Make sure you're attempting to work the previous pillars into your life first. But if you're ready for Pillar Six, it's time to get moving…physically that is!

A *couch potato* is defined by *Merriam-Webster.com* as a "lazy and inactive person; especially one who spends a great deal of time watching television."[8] That was the definition of me a little over two years ago after my injury. As you know, I have since embarked on a journey to wellness. And now it's your turn!

Looking back, I really began attempting to increase movement about a year after my injury. Because of my headaches and balance issues, I unfortunately have an issue with many of the types of exercise I did prior to my injury, and I haven't done well because I was looking at things all wrong. I thought if I couldn't exercise the "right" way, there was no point in doing anything. And, truthfully, I got a little bit lazy.

But what is the "right" way to exercise?

Good news—there isn't just one! The four categories of exercise

I want to discuss are endurance, strength, balance, and flexibility. Having a mix of all four is the best thing to do, but we will start with baby steps. First, I'll describe those four categories, then we can discuss how to easily add them into your routine.

ENDURANCE

Endurance exercise is the activity that will burn fat, also known by most as cardio. Such exercise includes brisk walking, jogging, doing yardwork, dancing, swimming, biking, rowing, using the elliptical, hiking, and playing sports such as football, soccer, basketball, or tennis. You may already be doing some type of endurance activity. If you are not, then the recommendation is to start off simple.

When I do any endurance exercise, I try to wear my smartwatch because it helps me to know how far I have gone, how long it has taken me, and where my heart rate lies in the targeted ranges (we will discuss this later). If you can't buy a smartwatch, a Fitbit or other off brand may be a better option. Or you can get a pedometer if you're only initially walking. (They are fairly inexpensive.)

I am sure you have heard that you should walk 10,000 steps daily. That is a good goal for most adults. Yet if you're fit and used to moving or have an active job, you may need more steps daily. If you are sedentary both at home and at work, 10,000 steps may be too many to begin. We'll strategize later how to work endurance exercise into your routine appropriately and at a pace that's comfortable for you.

STRENGTH

The second category of exercise is strength training, which is a necessary evil. Yes, I called it evil because I have always dreaded this type of exercise. I have always had a small upper body and since my shoulder surgery in early 2018, I have had right shoulder pain no matter what I do. Without strengthening your muscles, though, you cannot maximize fat-burning. More muscle equals more need to burn fat as you are exercising. Also even doing just body weight strength training regularly improves bone density and can decrease risk for osteoporosis later in life.

Strength training can include the use of weights, resistance bands, using objects at home (cans from the pantry), or using your own body weight. Weight or resistance training should be done at least twice weekly. There are many simple exercises that can be added to your routine, depending on where you need to focus. More details to come!

BALANCE

Balance exercise. Oh boy! This is one type where I still struggle. Prior to my injury hot yoga was one of my favorite things to do. I went to a little studio not far from my house, and it was the most amazing workout without feeling like a workout. I was relaxed when I finished and felt great. Then the next day I had that "hurts so good" feeling— you know the one that aches a little letting you know you worked out but not bad enough to really cause pain.

Yoga, whether done in a normal environment or in a hot room, is very beneficial for balance. It can also fit into strength training, flexibility, or endurance, depending on the type of yoga done. Depending on who you ask, there are anywhere from 5 to 8 types of yoga. I have really only practiced two—hatha and vinyasa—so I will discuss those.

Hatha yoga is a well-known type of yoga taught in many gyms and yoga studios. It's easy for beginners and teaches the importance of breathing and how to focus on the breath as you move through the different poses. Vinyasa yoga is a more dynamic yoga with continuous movement through different poses. It's for a more experienced person because it has a quicker pace. The studio where I practiced did classes of both of the types of yoga described above, but with the room set at 104°F.

Initially after my injury I couldn't keep my balance on level ground, let alone trying to do any exercise. I still have not tried yoga, and it has been over two years. I am slowly working other things into my routine, though. Believe it or not, working in a swimming pool is great to help improve balance. Some gyms or pools offer water aerobics classes, and those would be beneficial for balance, strengthening, and endurance.

Another type of exercise that can improve balance is tai chi. I have never personally practiced tai chi. It is a form of dynamic exercise but is at a slower and relaxed pace. It can benefit all four of the different categories listed here and can be altered for any level from beginner to advanced.

FLEXIBILITY

Flexibility is something many of us have issues with. Remember when you were a kid and could contort your body into random positions? Not anymore. Yoga and tai chi are both great exercises to help with flexibility and so is just simple stretching.

Working any of these categories into your routine can be helpful, and each person will need to work on different things. Some of us need to work on them all. If you're not currently doing any movement, discuss a plan with your medical provider before beginning to ensure you do not injure yourself. Starting slowly is okay!

MY MOVEMENT JOURNEY

I was in a better place pre-injury. Now I have some trouble doing certain things. I was able to slowly work my way back, but I am clearly nowhere near the end of my journey. How do I know?

Recently I was doing yard work with my husband and my max heart rate read by my smartwatch was 173 beats per minute (bpm). What? That is crazy! Maybe that is why I had to sit down and take a break a few times.

When talking about movement and exercise, one thing we should discuss is heart rate zones. Your maximum heart rate is about 220 minus your age. Mine is 179 bpm (i.e., 220 minus 41). There are 5 Heart Rate Zones.

- Zone 1 (*very* light physical activity such as walking) is 50–60% of maximum heart rate.
- Zone 2 (light physical activity) is 60–70% of maximum heart rate.
- Zone 3 (moderate physical activity) is 70–80% of maximum heart rate.
- Zone 4 (vigorous physical activity) is 80–90% of maximum heart rate.
- Zone 5 (extremely vigorous physical activity) is 90–100% of maximum heart rate. It's not recommended you exercise in the maximum zone.

The best zones to try to be in during any physical activity are Zones 1 through 3.

These zones allow you to be in the range of 50 to 80% of your target heart rate.

Looking back at my heart rate during my day of activity working in the yard, it was 96% of my maximum heart rate. It's so hard to believe it was that high. I was not doing anything that physical. I was trimming crepe myrtle bushes, and carrying and piling the branches. It should not have been that elevated. Looking back at this, I need to do more light or moderate physical activity in order to get myself back in shape.

To work activities into my schedule, I'll continue increasing my walking and rowing machine slowly while monitoring my heart rate. I will continue my lightweight training with resistance bands and small dumbbells. I try to alternate my days doing these and add in some balance and stretching on all days.

I'm no fitness coach or personal trainer, and some of you may have routines that work for you. This book is really reaching out to those of you who need motivation and help because you aren't sure where or how to start. I am trying to meet everyone where they are.

HOW TO ADD MOVEMENT SLOWLY

Here are ways you can increase your movement if you have a sedentary life or significant injury.

I. Start with finding out how many steps you take in a day by using a pedometer or smartwatch/Fitbit, etc. Then try to increase your number of steps. For example, if you regularly walk approximately 3,000 steps daily, try to increase your steps to 4,000 daily for a week, then 5,000 daily the next week, and so on. Initially start slowly walking, but then speed your pace to keep your heartrate in Zones 1 to 3 (50 to 80% of maximum heartrate). If your heart rate gets into zone 4 slow down. If you drop below 50% of your maximum, speed up.

2. If you have never weight trained, start with trying to do a wall pushup instead of a regular pushup, or by using 1-pound weights for a weight routine. If you have no weights, grab a can of vegetables out of the pantry. Remember more repetitions done properly are better than improper form with a heavier weight. If you need help with form or ideas of routines to do, go to my website *https://www.hot-mess-to-wellness.com/*.

3. If you have never worked on balance, start by just trying to lift a foot off the ground. How long could you stand on one foot? If you couldn't, use a chair or the wall initially to brace yourself. Then try multiple times daily to see if you can increase the amount of time.

4. If you have little to no flexibility, the best way to increase your flexibility is repetition. Sitting with legs fully extended, try to reach the farthest point on your legs. If you cannot reach your toes, it's okay. Strive to reach them multiple times daily. Remember repetition is key.

Here are ways you can increase your movement if you have a more active lifestyle.

1. Do a walk to jog/run routine sometimes known as a couch to 5K plan. Start off simple by just walking. Walk 30 minutes every day. I usually take one day a week off to rest. If every day is too much, start every other day. When you can walk consistently nonstop for 30 minutes, start jogging during the last 30 seconds of every 5 minutes. When you can do that consistently for 2 or 3

days, increase to the last minute of every 5 minutes. Try to keep your heartrate within Zones 1 to 3 (50 to 80% of maximum heartrate) as you increase from walking to jogging.

This is the routine my physical therapist had me doing. It really helped my physical and mental health because it was doable.

- (Walk 4:30, Jog 30 seconds) x 6 repetitions
- (Walk 4 min, Jog 1 min) x 6 repetitions
- (Walk 3:30, Jog 1:30 min) x 6 repetitions
- (Walk 3 min, Jog 2 min) x 6 repetitions
- (Walk 2:30, Jog 2:30 min) x 6 repetitions
- (Walk 2 min, Jog 3 min) x 6 repetitions
- (Walk 1:30, Jog 3:30 min) x 6 repetitions
- (Walk 1 min, Jog 4 min) x 6 repetitions
- (Walk 30 seconds, Jog 4:30 min) x 6 repetitions
- Run entire 30 minutes

2. Use bands or dumbbells to do a workout routine. You can slowly increase as you improve. You should always start with 10 to 15 repetitions of each exercise in 3 sets. Rest between sets. If a weight feels too heavy or you notice your form is incorrect, choose the next size down in weight.

As an example, let's say you are doing dumbbell curls. Start with the appropriate weight—one that's not too heavy. Remember that more reps at lighter weight is better than poor form and hurting yourself using a weight that is too heavy.

Also, if you are looking for lean muscle mass, more reps and lighter weight is better and if you are looking to bulk up more weight with fewer reps is better.

- Start with 10-15 repetitions, rest 1 minute.
- Do 10-15 more repetitions, rest 1 minute.
- Do 10-15 more repetitions.

If you feel the weight is not challenging you, choose the next heavier weight.

3. Join a yoga, tai chi, or water aerobics class to work on both balance and flexibility.

As far as movement, I don't have specific work out plans because I feel everyone needs a plan unique to their journey. I do have a few more ways you can work the four different types of exercise into your routine, go to *https://www.hot-mess-to-wellness.com/* for more details.

Chapter 8

FINDING THE SUPPORT YOU NEED FOR YOUR JOURNEY

"ONLY YOU CAN START YOUR JOURNEY, BUT THAT DOESN'T MEAN YOU ARE ALONE. SURROUND YOURSELF WITH POSITIVE PEOPLE AND LET GO OF NEGATIVITY." –AMANDA ZEINE

We've finally reached Pillar Seven. This is probably the most important pillar because we all need someone to lean on at some point, especially in the beginning as you start your journey from hot mess to wellness.

To take this guide and truly put it into practice and create these healthy habits, it will take repetition and dedication. Having support gives you accountability and helps you to stick with it. When I attempted to work on my health in the beginning, I felt alone. Even with my supportive family, the Warrior Transition Unit with their adaptive reconditioning program, and my friends, I felt alone. I thought no one really understood where I was on this journey and how I felt.

I was sitting alone in the dark, ordering comfort food through delivery apps. I was depressed and unsure what to do. I gained weight, then became even more depressed. I was unable to function as I had prior to the injury. The more I tried to lose weight, the more depressed I became because even if I lost weight, I would then gain it all back. Sometimes I gained even more. I was truly a *Hot Mess*.

What was the problem? There were many. First of all, I felt alone when I wasn't. Many of us suffer in this way. I am writing this book, so you know you are not the only one suffering.

I had family, friends, and an amazing healthcare team that was there to support me in every way. I just needed to reach out. Stop and think about it. Are you married? Reach out to your spouse. Talk to them and explain your situation. Let your voice be heard.

Do you have family nearby or even just a phone call away? Reach out because chances are they understand what you are going through.

Do you have friends, coworkers, acquaintances at church? Reach out. You would be amazed how many people have the same fears and anxieties about life.

If you feel you have no one to reach out to or are afraid to reach out, then join me. Part of my goal in writing this book was to form a community for like-minded people because we all need accountability partners.

During the darkest part of my journey, I felt isolated, as if there was no one who could understand my situation. I looked for self-help books and groups. There are groups on Facebook and other blogs on the internet, but I felt many of those did not reach out to the average person and meet them where they are.

Since I began writing this book, I have found a few groups similar to what I am trying to establish. But I've designed a group that truly meets you where you are right now in your journey. Whether that's just starting out, feeling lost, ready for the next pillar, etc., you'll find a welcoming and inspiring community.

Visit my website to see my favorite links, read my blog, even contact me directly with questions or suggestions. Once you join the community, there is a discussion forum, and you can look for an accountability partner or partners. We should all be working to lift one another up and support one another in this journey.

This book is just the beginning of my journey. I hope to reach many and help you see that you are perfect the way you are. But, if you want to feel better, you can take that one step to join me and get started on your own life-changing journey. I know how you feel and want you to know there are many who share in your feelings.

As you travel your journey from hot mess to wellness, you may not always succeed the first time. That's okay! Get up and try again. You may also have to revisit a chapter to refresh yourself down the road and that's okay, too. If you find it impossible to follow the exact recommendations I make, alter it to fit your lifestyle. There is not a one-size-fits-all solution to better health. I want you to understand, though, that if you want to be healthier that there is a way, and I want to help motivate you to take that first step. Join me. We are all on this journey together.

After writing this book, I am excited to help others. I hope to start a book series for children introducing them to the world of yummy fruits and veggies, discussing issues they face in the "tween" years, and showing them it can be fun to do things other than play video games! I envision a possible book similar to this geared toward teens and even one geared toward parents, instructing them on how to bring health into their children's lives. If you have any ideas, please join my website at *https://www.hot-mess-to-wellness.com/* and share them with me.

ACKNOWLEDGEMENTS

I would like to extend a huge thank you to my family and friends for supporting me through my initial journey of becoming a physician in the United States Army. It was a long journey, and many sacrificed, including my daughter who has endured many hardships. She has amazing resilience, and I love her and thank her more than I could ever say.

I would also like to thank my family and friends for supporting me through my low points after my injury. An extra thank you to my husband who is my rock, and to his family for caring for me and physically supporting me through my recovery and the writing of this book.

To my family (including my best friend Manda Jo), thank you for always being there, although at a distance, for encouragement.

I would also like to thank Self-Publishing School (SPS) and my coaches Kerk and Brett. Without SPS, I would not have had the knowledge or courage to publish this book.

Finally, I would like to thank my editor Val Cervarich who was patient with me as a new writer, and Danijela and Mariska at Cutting Edge Studios for their amazing cover design and formatting help.

REFERENCES

American Academy of Sleep Medicine, last modified 2021, *https://aasm.org/*

Bulsiewicz, Will. *Fiber Fueled: The Plant Based Gut Health Program for Losing Weight, Restoring Health, and Optimizing Your Microbiome.* New York: Penguin Random House, 2020. Penguin audio, ed. 7 hr., 11 min.

Centers for Disease Control and Prevention (CDC), Division of Nutrition, Physical Activity, and Obesity, National Center for Chronic Disease Prevention and Health Promotion, "Adult Obesity Facts," Overweight & Obesity, last modified June 7, 2021, *https://www.cdc.gov/obesity/data/adult.html.*

Drake, Christopher, Timothy Roehrs, John Shambroom, and Thomas Roth. "Caffeine effects on sleep taken 0, 3, or 6 hours before going to bed." *Journal of Clinical Sleep Medicine* 9, no. 11 (2013): 1195–1200.

Hyman, Mark. *Food: What the Heck Should I Eat?* Read by Mark Hyman. New York: Hachette Book Group Audio, 2018. Hachette audio ed., 10 hr., 21 min.

Merriam-Webster.com, s.v. "couch potato,"
https://www.merriam-webster.com/dictionary/couch%20potato.
Merriam-Webster.com, s.v. "mindfulness,"
https://www.merriam-webster.com/dictionary/mindfulness.

Ohayon, Maurice M., Mary A. Carskadon, Christian Guilleminault, and Michael V. Vitiello. "Meta-analysis of quantitative sleep parameters from childhood to old age in healthy individuals: developing normative sleep values across the human lifespan." *Sleep* 27, no. 7 (2004): 1255–1273.

Simopoulos, Artemis P. "An increase in the omega-6/omega-3 fatty acid ratio increases the risk for obesity." *Nutrients* 8, no. 3 (2016): 128.

US Department of Agriculture, "MyPlate," *https://www.myplate.gov/.*

Thank You for Reading My Book!

I need your input to make future books better.
Please leave an honest review on Amazon letting me
know what you thought of the book.

Thanks so much!

Amanda

ENDNOTES

1 Merriam-Webster.com, s.v. "mindfulness," *https://www.merriam-webster.com/dictionary/mindfulness.*

2 American Academy of Sleep Medicine, last modified 2021, *https://aasm.org/*; Maurice M. Ohayon, Mary A. Carskadon, Christian Guilleminault, and Michael V. Vitiello. "Meta-analysis of quantitative sleep parameters from childhood to old age in healthy individuals: developing normative sleep values across the human lifespan." *Sleep* 27, no. 7 (2004): 1255–1273.

3 Christopher Drake, Timothy Roehrs, John Shambroom, and Thomas Roth, "Caffeine effects on sleep taken 0, 3, or 6 hours before going to bed," *Journal of Clinical Sleep Medicine* 9, no. 11 (2013): 1195–1200.

4 Centers for Disease Control and Prevention (CDC), Division of Nutrition, Physical Activity, and Obesity, National Center for Chronic Disease Prevention and Health Promotion, "Adult Obesity Facts," Overweight & Obesity, last modified June 7, 2021, *https://www.cdc.gov/obesity/data/adult.html.*

5 US Department of Agriculture, "MyPlate," *https://www.myplate.gov/.*

6 Mark Hyman, *Food: What the Heck Should I Eat?* read by Mark Hyman, New York: Hachette Book Group Audio, 2018, Hachette audio ed., 10 hr., 21 min.; Will Bulsiewicz, *Fiber Fueled: The Plant Based Gut Health Program for Losing Weight, Restoring Health, and Optimizing Your Microbiome*, New York: Penguin Random House, 2020, Penguin

audio, ed. 7 hr., 11 min.

7Artemis P. Simopoulos, "An increase in the omega-6/omega-3 fatty acid ratio increases the risk for obesity," *Nutrients* 8, no. 3 (2016): 128.

8Merriam-Webster.com, s.v. "couch potato,"

https://www.merriam-webster.com/dictionary/couch%20potato.

Made in the USA
Monee, IL
04 January 2022

87934628R00056